PROMOTING PARTNERSHIP FOR HEALTH

Service user and carer involvement in education for health and social care

Dedication

In the course of our involvement with service user and carer participation in university settings we have lost some valued friends and colleagues along the way. We dedicate this book to those individuals whose untimely deaths mean they will not see this book but who nevertheless contributed greatly to it.

Les Collier
Lillian Hughes
Eileen Johnson
Ian Light
Sandy Richardson

All have in their own way supported us, loved and cared for us, challenged us, been kind to us, made us laugh and inspired us to see this project through. They will be sadly missed and fondly remembered.

PROMOTING PARTNERSHIP FOR HEALTH

Service user and carer involvement in education for health and social care

Mick McKeown
Principal Lecturer
Mental Health Division
School of Nursing & Caring Science
University of Central Lancashire, Preston & Comensus

Lisa Malihi-Shoja
Comensus Co-ordinator
Comensus, Faculty of Health
University of Central Lancashire, Preston

Soo Downe
Professor of Midwifery Studies
School of Public Health & Clinical Sciences
University of Central Lancashire, Preston

Supporting the Comensus Writing Collective

http://www.uclan.ac.uk/health/about_health/health_comensus.php

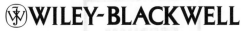
WILEY-BLACKWELL
A John Wiley & Sons, Ltd., Publication

CAIPE

This edition first published 2010
© 2010 Blackwell Publishing Ltd

Blackwell Publishing was acquired by John Wiley & Sons in February 2007. Blackwell's publishing programme has been merged with Wiley's global Scientific, Technical, and Medical business to form Wiley-Blackwell.

Registered office
John Wiley & Sons Ltd, The Atrium, Southern Gate, Chichester, West Sussex, PO19 8SQ, United Kingdom

Editorial offices
9600 Garsington Road, Oxford, OX4 2DQ, United Kingdom
2121 State Avenue, Ames, Iowa 50014-8300, USA

For details of our global editorial offices, for customer services and for information about how to apply for permission to reuse the copyright material in this book please see our website at www.wiley.com/wiley-blackwell.

Library of Congress Cataloging-in-Publication Data

McKeown, Mick.
  Service user & carer involvement in education for health & social care / Mick McKeown, Lisa Malihi-Shoja, Soo Downe, supporting the Comensus Writing Collective.
    p. ; cm. – (Promoting partnership for health)
  Includes bibliographical references.
    ISBN 978-1-4051-8432-8 (hardback : alk. paper)   1. Academic medical centers.   2. Public health.
3. Social service.   4. Community health services.   I. Malihi-Shoja, Lisa.   II. Downe, Soo.   III. Title.
IV. Title: Service user and carer involvement in education for health and social care.   V. Series: Promoting partnership for health.
  [DNLM: 1. Health Education.   2. Community Health Services–organization & administration.
3. Community-Institutional Relations.   4. Consumer Participation.   5. Health Policy.   6. Social Work–education. WA 18 M478s 2010]
  RA966.M35 2010
  362.1–dc22

                                                                                    2009049071

A catalogue record for this book is available from the British Library.

Set in 10/12.5 pt Palatino by Aptara® Inc., New Delhi, India
Printed in Singapore by Markono Print Media Pte Ltd

1   2010

Contents

Promoting Partnership for Health

This book is one of six in the 'Promoting Partnership for Health' series published by Wiley in association with the Centre for the Advancement of Interprofessional Education (CAIPE). They address partnership to improve the health and well being of individuals, families and communities from different but complementary perspectives.

Three of the books focus on partnership in practice. Geoff Meads and John Ashworth demonstrate how collaboration has proved critical to effective implementation of health care reforms in many countries around the world. John Glasby and Helen Dickinson assemble authoritative sources from Australia, Europe and North America to understand integrated care from many different angles. Scott Reeves and his colleagues contribute a rigorous and wide-ranging critique of interprofessional teamwork informed by evidence and theory and within a robust framework.

Two of the books focus on interprofessional education as a means to promote collaborative practice. Hugh Barr and colleagues embed findings from a systematic review. Della Freeth and her colleagues marry that evidence with their experience to assist all who are engaged in developing, delivering and evaluating interprofessional education programmes.

Partnership between service providers and users is a recurrent theme throughout the series, a message reinforced persuasively in this book which demonstrates dividends for all concerned when service users and carers are fully engaged in preparing future practitioners for partnership in practice.

Hugh Barr
Series Editor

The books in the series:

Barr, H., Koppel, I., Reeves, S., Hammick, M. & Freeth, D. (2005) Effective interprofessional education: Argument, assumption and evidence.

Freeth, D., Hammick, M., Reeves. S., Koppel, I, & Barr, H. (2005) Effective interprofessional education: Development, delivery and evaluation.

Meads, G, & Ashcroft, J. with Barr, H., Scott, R, & Wild, A. (2005) The case for collaboration in health and social care.

Glasby, J. & Dickinson, H. (2009) International perspectives on health and social care.

Reeves S, Lewin S, Espin S & Zwarenstein M (2010) Interprofessional teamwork for health and social care.

McKeown, M., Malihi Shoja, L. & Downe, S. supporting the Comensus Writing Collective (2010) Service user and carer involvement in education for health and social care

Foreword: Strike up the Band!

Kathryn Church* with David Reville**
*Associate Professor and **Instructor, School of Disability Studies,
Ryerson University, Toronto, Canada.

The thing you've got to learn is not to be afraid of it.
(Robbie Robertson, *The Band*)

This book makes a unique contribution to the international body of literature on "user involvement." [1] A significant portion of the text documents what happened in a single university when service users and carers and allied academics worked together to bring their lived experience to the teaching of health and social care. Until now, services and systems have been the major arena for practice, policy, analysis and writing on this topic. At long last, a tipping point into the field of education as a fresh site for activity. Thus, there is much to celebrate.

We celebrate the practice that lies at the heart of this volume. The knowing revealed here, layer by layer, is not your standard academic fare: detached, abstract, speculative. Rather, this knowing is grounded in direct engagement with a tangible project – the initiative called Comensus – and the dilemmas that emerged from that work: day by day, year to year. Here we are offered real people, their actions and interactions in place and time. Situated in social and political context, these particularities resonate widely – across an ocean, in our case. In the sentences assembled, as well as the tensions that run silently between the lines, we recognize the familiar world of our own complex struggles.

We celebrate the array of players whose efforts made both Comensus and this volume possible. As veterans of participatory projects, including research, we know how difficult working across difference can be. In Canada, the lure of grants for community-university partnerships has been strong over the past few years. But rarely do these arrangements extend beyond the terms of the funding. Faced with the challenging "between-ness" of collaborative scholarship – neither this nor that, here nor there, me nor thee – the Comensus players stayed the course. Their grit is our gain as this account disrupts and breaks open the traditional separations between these worlds.

---

[1] In these remarks, we embrace the term "user involvement" while we also use the following: consumer, consumer participation, psychiatric survivors, "mad", and Mad Studies. All of these words are actively "at play" in the mental health and university worlds in Toronto.

We celebrate the writing itself. The literature on participatory action research is thick with suggestions for how participants should work collectively to shape major phases of the process (Mental Health Recovery Study Group, 2009). It is less than forthcoming, however, on how to produce a participatory text; participation often breaks down at the point of writing. Not so with this book. From the moment you crack its pages, you realize that you are reading something different. You anticipate a dominant author and discover a generous collectivity. You search for a status hierarchy and find a level playing field. You expect singularity and are surprised by multiplicity. You steel yourself for turgidity and relax into welcoming prose.

On what basis do we strike up this "band"? For 25 years, David and I have been working on, observing, thinking through and writing about user involvement. We embody a case study that ranges across community, government and university sites from local to international levels. Our first project was a national policy initiative of the Canadian Mental Health Association. From 1984–1988, I staffed the volunteer committee that directed what came to be known as "Building a Framework for Support." Through research, documentation and a couple of daring experiments, this group put consumer participation on the mental health "map" of every province in Canada. David was our first consumer representative, and, later, the first consumer member of the organization's national board of directors.

David: I was elected to Toronto City Council in 1980 as part of a reform movement that emphasized citizen participation. Open about having a mental health history, I was a member of one of Canada's first mental patients' associations (Reville, 1981). My political base, however, came from work in educational politics and poverty law. When the Mayor set up a task force on discharged psychiatric patients, it was no stretch for me to insist that he appoint people we now describe as "experts by experience". When I introduced Pat Capponi, a recently discharged psychiatric patient and fierce advocate for better housing for her "folks", to Dr. Reva Gerstein, the chair of the task force, I did not know what I had wrought. The alliance that developed between the two women produced significant and long-lasting change. I didn't know that "user participation" was a "thing" until Kathryn recruited me for the policy committee she staffed at CMHA National. By then I had moved on to provincial politics and I took with me a growing reputation as a user who was going to participate come what may. In my second term in the legislature, I was my party's health critic so I was able to put mental health on the agenda much more often than was usual.

Trying to shift an entire organization – its language, structures and practices – is an enormous challenge on many fronts. I soon discovered a huge gap between my training in psychology and the skills required for national community development. Of necessity, I became a practitioner/learner (for lack of a better term), someone engaged in trial-and-error learning-by-doing that was always, hopefully, just-in-time. David mentored me. I relied on his advice to navigate the turbulence that bubbled up when our attempts to involve new players met with organizational resistance. Through him, I came to understand that our vision for change had to go beyond better service planning. It had to engage the democratic agenda of other social movements. It had to become political.

David: As a "leftie" with community organizing experience, I was shocked at how a-political CMHA was. I was shocked, too, at its tolerance of the glacial pace of change. As a city councillor, I'd begged city bureaucrats to open abandoned buildings so that homeless men and women could get in out of the cold; my executive assistant and I cut up sheets of bubble wrap so that they wouldn't have to sleep on bare floors. And here comes the Canadian Mental Health Association wanting to "scan the external environment"?

CMHA's policy agenda was puzzling, too. The notion that a person with mental health issues needed the support not just of the mental health system but of community agencies, families, friends and peers seemed to me so self-evident that I didn't understand why anybody had taken the trouble to put it into a book. But as I travelled around the country telling the "Framework for Support" story, I began to realize that (a) the story wasn't self-evident and (b) that being a part of national organization provided real opportunities to showcase the "user voice". Were it not for my connection to CMHA, I don't think I would have been invited to the Common Concerns conference. Invitation in hand, I called Kathryn; I needed a paper on user involvement.

"Common Concerns" was held at the University of Sussex, England, in 1988. That international event was likely the first of its kind: a landmark in the "user movement" worldwide. To the assembled company, David delivered our co-authored paper on user involvement in Canada. It was a "work in progress", we argued, pointing to examples of member control over self-help organizations and housing cooperatives, coalitions for supportive legislation and partnerships for progressive policy development. An increasing number of professionals were realizing that they had to learn "not to be afraid of it."

After leaving the mental health association, our collaboration revolved around my doctoral studies. As I embraced sociology, David connected me to the psychiatric survivor leaders whose stories and politics constituted a standpoint for my research. His legislative challenges to the provincial government sparked a series of regional policy consultations that became the lively ground of my formal inquiry. I had a seat in the front row from which to observe the profound "unsettlement" that occurred as people who had been diagnosed and treated by a service system sought to find their way as "knowers" in its governance. The process was emotional and disturbing – a far cry from the cool rationality of "democratic representation." My analysis surfaced the "breaking down/breaking through" of forms and relations, discourses and practices that comes with "passionate participation" (Barnes, 2008). One sharp edge of my personal breakdown was the split in my learning between the university's demands for proper scientific stance and form, and psychiatric survivor demands for authentic presence and activist engagement (Church, 1993; 1995).

In the 1990s, a conservative government took power in Ontario. The years that followed were not kind to participatory initiatives of any sort. David and I were each compelled to reorganize our paid work. He left politics to lead the new Advocacy Commission of Ontario – and to preside over its demise when it was axed by the province. I built a practice as an independent researcher working primarily for psychiatric survivor organizations doing community economic development – an activity favoured by funders of that period. I organized a series of small participatory studies and wrote plain language reports on survivor-run community businesses. These projects demonstrated the flip side of user involvement. Psychiatric survivor organizations set the terms for the work and controlled the funds; I was contractual labour. And while that arrangement clarified our power relations, I grew troubled over identity politics and the uncertain or fleeting impact that community-based research had on policy. Privately, I yearned for greater intellectual freedom.

David: Involvement with CMHA both nationally and internationally turned me into a kind of poster boy for user participation. Over time, however, my focus shifted to policy and program development designed to create and sustain user-led initiatives. Some of the most successful user-led initiatives were – and remain – community-based businesses. For the employees of such businesses, it is participation by people who are not users that is contentious. The politics of user participation began to change in the early 90s. More and more activists began to identify as survivors rather than users and began to reject offers to merely participate. One user-led organization now feels sufficiently comfortable in its own skin that it is partnering with service providers; it continues to provide social recreation opportunities for its members but also is part of a mental health system program that seeks to keep users out of the justice system. The leadership of another user-led organization has linked up with anti-poverty activists; one of its members has appointed to a panel to advise the government on a review of social assistance.

By the end of the decade, David and I were both working as consultants within Toronto's community and social services sector. Occasionally, we overlapped into shared projects such as providing advice on the production of the film titled "Working Like Crazy", and sustaining the international discussion generated by its dissemination. We were figuring out how to practice in an altered social and political environment, one in which traditional forums for gathering, exchanging views and creating action had been smudged or erased. We were learning to make do with "the remains of the day": with smaller projects and more fragmentation, with less funding and a more meager array of democratic tools.

In 2002, I joined the School of Disability Studies at Ryerson University. I have since become a tenured faculty member, making the tricky cross-over from mental health to disability writ-large, and expanding my considerations of difference and inclusion in theory and everyday life. Captured by the escalating demands of teaching, research and service, my wisest move was to draw David into the mix. He joined the program in 2004, initially as guest lecturer and co-instructor, and later as a regular, part-time instructor. For seven years, he has been openly and productively "mad" in the academy.

David: I'm excited to bring user knowledge to 330 students a year; that's how many students enroll in A History of Madness. As gratified as I am about the number, I am even more delighted that the students come from all five university faculties. Students from, say, mechanical engineering, psychology, image arts and information technology management may give a group presentation. My other mad course, Mad People's History, is now online, available to anybody with access to a computer. The first module includes a video in which 12 user activists describe how and why they self-label. The final module asks the question: whither mad studies? This book will provide a foundation on which to build a good part of the answer.

This university adventure looks to be the final iteration of our long grappling with user involvement. It has provoked a number of questions. Are people with mental health histories "experts by experience" only in matters of illness and treatment? Is creating awareness through personal stories the only result we seek from their involvement in the university? David's expertise begins with his mental health history but his fuller contribution is to retrieve the history of a people – a rich and complex body of knowledge that challenges the psychiatric worldview. On the flip side, by weighting "experience" do we devalue the expertise that academics spend years developing? And, from a different angle, are academics experts only with respect to credentialed content in their particular disciplines? Are their "lived experiences" as multi-dimensional human characters never entered into the classroom? There is a personal story – a political autobiography – at the core of my pedagogy. In Disability Studies, I am not alone in insisting upon its relevance as knowledge. And, finally, given the continual reshaping of universities as institutions, can we continue to view them as public institutions? How will user involvement play against the intensification of corporate involvement and funding? Our program has been on the cutting edge of this question for a decade.

David: As we start the second decade of a new century, user involvement is making a comeback in Canada. The newly-created Mental Health Commission is trumpeting the amount of user involvement in its deliberations. An all-user consulting team is crisscrossing the country scouting out user participation wherever it may be found. The Commission has funded a huge research study examining the relationship of homelessness and mental health; the studies at the five project sites include varying amounts of user involvement.

Given the broad relevance of these matters, this book makes a timely appearance. We know that it will be valued – read, quoted, cited, critiqued, even emulated – well beyond the borders of its origins. We congratulate everyone who contributed. Where power relations are deeply entrenched, it takes real courage to venture something new.

Selected References

Barnes, M. 2008. Passionate participation: Emotional experiences and expressions in deliberative forum. *Critical Social Policy, 28* (461–481).

Church, K. 1995. *Forbidden Narratives: Critical Autobiography as Social Science.* Amsterdam: International Publishers Distributors. Reprinted by Routledge, London.

Church, K. 1993. *Breaking down/Breaking through: Multi-Voiced Narratives on Psychiatric Survivor Participation in Ontario's Community Mental Health System.* Doctoral Dissertation, Ontario Institute for Studies in Education, University of Toronto.

Church, K. & Reville, D. 1990. User involvement in mental health services in Canada. In *Report of 'Common Concerns' - International Conference on User Involvement in Mental Health Services.* England: East Sussex Social Services, Brighton Health Authority and MIND.

Mental Health Recovery Study Research Group. 2009. *Mental Health "Recovery:" Users and Refusers.* Toronto: Wellesley Institute. Toronto: Ryerson-RBC Institute for Disability Studies Research and Education.

Reville, D. 1981. Don't Spyhole Me, (Hospital Journal) *Phoenix Rising: The Voice of the Psychiatrized.* Vol. 2, No. 1 (Spring 1981 – pp. 18–41) http://psat.hostrator.com/pheonix/pheonix_21.pdf

The Comensus Writing Collective: Notes on Authorship

Rather than producing a standard edited text, we have aimed to write a collectively produced multi-authored book.

For the bulk of the book we have practised a process of collective writing, supported by a series of writing team meetings and other individual and peer support, such that authorship of the text is shared. Initial meetings discussed the potential structure and content of the book, agreeing the sort of material we might cover, and the different ways in which individuals might wish to be involved. Different people have facilitated the writing of different chapters, and these have progressed via an iterative process of drafting, peer feedback, and re-drafting. Our notion of authorship involves creative approaches for including the contributions of those individuals who have less experience of writing for publication. Some people have written sections of text, of varying lengths, in more or less a standard approach to writing. Others have preferred to look at drafts of emerging text and bring in their contribution based upon reflecting on these as a starting point. Some people have preferred to sit down individually and talk through their ideas for material to be included, with another person making notes and attempting to draft these out, before passing back to the originator for approval. On other occasions, this sort of thing has been accomplished collectively in group meetings.

Once we were at the stage of having completed drafts of chapters, these were circulated collectively for critical feedback and comments. A smaller group of people was responsible for collating the results of this critical reading process, and incorporating changes into the draft manuscript. A number of us have also contributed quotes which appear at chapter heads, connecting personal reflections on involvement with the thematic content of the specific chapters.

Of necessity, certain chapters have been solely written by named authors, and some sections of other chapters are clearly the contributions of other named individuals. In these instances, authors are explicitly identified at the chapter head, or at the point in the text where their contribution comes in. Though this may seem to go against the grain of our philosophy for a completely collectively written text, the rationale for this emerged out of discussions in the collective.

Our reasoning for a collectivised approach was in some way to shift from standard academic practice of attributing authorship and editorship. We felt that some traditional approaches were less democratic than they might be, and did not always adequately reflect the multiplicity of ways in which contributions to ideas and writings can be made, especially given that our starting point for the book was nested in a participatory action research project. For these reasons, the idea of collective authorship, with all contributors to the collective given equal credit had much appeal within our group. In this sense, our approach is very much in line with the notion of a 'creative commons'.

This simple collective approach, however, runs the risk of devaluing input by individuals who have put a lot of effort into crafting their contribution, and wish to be identified with it. Hence, our decision to properly credit key portions of writing identifiably associated with single authors. These other authors are also credited more widely for other contributions to the collective enterprise elsewhere in the book. We haven't imposed an 'editorial voice' on contributions which are explicitly auto-biographical or describe examples from practice (see Cox et al., 2008). Editorial work was an integral part of collective discussions and the writing process, and not vested in any single individual.

The members of the collective are listed here in alphabetical order:

Waheda Ahmed (Comensus CIT & Preston Community Network)

Mahmud Amirat (Comensus Advisory Group & Preston Gujarat Muslim Welfare Society)

Jill Anderson (Lancaster University & mhhe)

Nurjahan Badat (Comensus CIT & parent carer)

Phil Blundell (University of Central Lancashire)

Carol Catterall-Maguire (Comensus community member)

Caroline Brown (Independent service user)

David Catherall (Comensus CIT)

Melanie Close (Comensus Advisory Group & Preston Disability Information Services Centre)

Les Collier (Comensus CIT & Preston Mental Health Service User Forum)

Anthony Conder (Comensus Advisory Group & Central Lancashire Primary Care Trust)

Rose Cork (Comensus CIT)

Pat Cox (University of Central Lancashire)

John Coxhead (Comensus CIT & Preston DISC)

Paul Dixon (Comensus CIT & REACT)

Soo Downe (Comensus/University of Central Lancashire)

Stephanie Doherty (Comensus CIT)

Joy Duxbury (University of Central Lancashire)

Chris Essen (University of Leeds)

Janet Garner (Comensus/University of Central Lancashire)

Michael Gardner (Comensus CIT)

Nigel Harrison (University of Central Lancashire)

Janice Hanson (Uniformed Services University of the Health Sciences, Bethesda, Maryland)

Michael Hellawell (University of Bradford)

Russell Hogarth (Comensus CIT & Preston SMILE)

Keith Holt (Comensus CIT & Giving Experience Meaning)

Robert Hopkins (Comensus CIT & Preston DISC)

Graham Hough (Comensus community member & Preston Mental Health Service User Forum)

Lillian Hughes (Comensus CIT)

Eileen Johnson (Comensus/University of Central Lancashire)

Fiona Jones (Comensus community member & Preston Mental Health Service User Forum)

Brenda Jules (Comensus CIT)

David Liberato (Comensus CIT)

Beth Lown (Mount Auburn Hospital, Cambridge, Massachusetts)

John Lunt (Comensus CIT & Preston Mental Health Service User Forum)

Farida Majumder (Comensus CIT & parent carer)

Ernie Mallen (Comensus CIT)

Lisa Malihi-Shoja (Comensus/University of Central Lancashire)

Marie Mather (Comensus Advisory Group & University of Central Lancashire)

Angela McCarthy-Grunwald (Comensus/University of Central Lancashire)

David McCollom (Comensus community member)

Mick McKeown (Comensus/University of Central Lancashire)

Phil McClenaghan (Comensus CIT)

Angela Melling (Comensus CIT & parent carer)

Bob Minto (Comensus Advisory Group & Central Lancashire Primary Care Trust)

Kate Murry (Comensus CIT & parent carer)

William Park (Independent service user & poet)

Hasumati Parmar (Comensus CIT & Preston Mental Health Service User Forum)

Jane Priestley (University of Bradford)

Phyllis Prior-Egerton (Comensus CIT & Transinclusion)

Sue Ramsdale (University of Central Lancashire)

Lou Rawcliffe (Comensus CIT)

Alan Simpson (City University, London)

Nat Solanki (Comensus CIT)

Helen Spandler (University of Central Lancashire)

Peter Sullivan (Comensus CIT & Preston Carers Centre)

Jacqui Vella (Comensus CIT & Preston Breathe Easy)

Sarah Whelan (Comensus CIT)

Grahame Wilding (Comensus CIT & Preston HIV Support Team)

Karen Wright (University of Central Lancashire)

The Comensus Writing Collective can be contacted via the Comensus web-pages:
http://www.uclan.ac.uk/health/about_health/health_comensus.php

Notes on Language

Our book is about the contribution made to universities by people who have experienced health and social care or who act in the role of informal carer. The language used to describe participants in these endeavours is sometimes controversial and contested. It is our experience not to take these matters for granted.

A focus on choice of terminology is, arguably, more important than idle curiosity or interest in changing fashions. A post-structuralist turn in social sciences suggests that language and discourse are not merely descriptive of objectively verifiable phenomena or social relations. Rather, language and terminology themselves are constitutive, bringing into being that which we recognise as real. The subjective positioning of the viewer or author is privileged in these accounts, and a plurality of ways of making sense of the social world is accepted. The use of different forms of language is often associated with prevailing power relations, with dominant discourses acting to limit or close down alternative or oppositional talk.

In an everyday sense these concerns are exemplified in the wider politics of user involvement in health and social care and, amongst other things, in the debate about use of terminology amongst professional disciplines and lay talk surrounding notions of so-called political correctness. Because ideologies and circumstances can change, individuals who use health and social care services find themselves constructed differently in language as time passes. Examples of this would be the predominance of the term *patient* in circumstances where medical power is in the ascendancy or the language of *consumers* and *clients* at times when individualistic, possibly market driven, ideologies challenged prevailing medical hegemony. Of course, such broad brush trends are complicated by other factors, not least the influence of diverse ideological standpoints or narratives across different health and social care disciplines at different moments in history.

On the face of it, it would seem that the terminology surrounding informal care, that is looking after someone else in an unpaid capacity, typically a relative, is much less contentious than the numerous appellations that have been afforded the role of recipient of formal, professionalised care services. The label carer can be accepted without too much fuss. Though the practice of caring can be associated with aspects of social disadvantage, the role is largely approved of in society. For others, the term 'carer' can be problematic, fore-grounding important socioeconomic and identity issues. The language used to describe people who make use of services, however, can at various junctures be implicitly or explicitly pejorative, demeaning and stigmatising. Different terms applied to this role or identity have appeal for some but not others, and it is very difficult to find a single term that is not flawed in some regard and is acceptable across the board. There are also some variations in use of terminology on an international scale, with slightly different descriptors for key lay participation roles in university settings. This latter point is addressed by the authors of chapter 4, who offer a glossary of some such terms in usage in the US.

Authors of a text which has to cover this territory, hence, are presented with an immediate dilemma over which terminology to favour. Apart from the politics and potential for causing offence to some of the readership we would hope to be interested in this book, there are also practical concerns around reading ease. The latter militate against chopping and changing terms throughout a text, or forever expanding one's descriptors to accommodate all possible nuances of meaning for any given context. This would include repeatedly pausing to explain the pros and cons, or exceptions to, particular terminology at different junctures in the narrative. Ultimately, there is also a need to choose a term that is meaningful to the readership, being instantly recognisable as the entity it is meant to signify. To a large extent this choice involves deciding upon one of the terms which has wide current use. Coining our own neologism would not work in this regard, and certainly couldn't be incorporated in the title of a book that was seeking a broad audience.

Over the years such terms as *patient, service user, consumer,* or *lay participant* have come in for different criticisms (see Beresford, 2005a; Deber et al., 2005). Similar debates surround the terminology of *disability* and *disabled people* (Swain et al., 2003). The language of *patient* is wrapped up in notions of passive subservience and deference to medical authority and variations on *client* and *consumer,* though in some respects an attempt to indicate greater personal agency, are redolent of a market driven ideology of consumerism that is anathema for some. The current policy vogue for public participation, at least at the level of rhetoric, does not on its own differentiate the particularities of engagement in health and social care from the generalities of the public at large. Terms deployed within the *user movement* that are relevant to our interests here, include *activist* and *survivor.* Despite the notion of activism appearing to often closely fit the behaviour of relevant participants engaged in universities and *community voluntarism,* many people do not recognise the term as fitting in with their view of themselves. The term *survivor* also lacks appeal for many such participants, and, in any event, can have a more recognisably general meaning than its specific use in *service user movement* culture.

In a research context, the notion of *participant* would seem to be superior to *subject,* or other previously relied on depersonalising terminology, including the not uncommon practice in earlier medical journals of describing people's *involvement* under the heading *materials and methods.*

In this book, we have used *service user* and *carer* in the absence of better terms. The term *service user* can be variously criticised, and Beresford (2005a) lists a number of shortcomings. These include disapproval for representing a degree of passivity in encounters with professionals and services, reducing identity to aspects of service usage alone, neglect of the reality that for some people there is a lack of choice in consumption of public services, or for some their use of services is compulsory, and, like all labels, there is a potential for the heterogeneity of personal experience to be obliterated in the homogenising effects of a single term to catch all. Others have objected to the potential for confusion with different notions of *user*, as in the argot of illicit drug use or the view of people as manipulative. There has been some disquiet that the term is perceived as lower status than other professional titles, and this has been noted in a university context by William Park (Chapter 10 this volume). The phraseology of *expert by experience* has been coined to counteract this sort of thing.

The term *service user* has, however, been adopted and employed for radical ends by some in the user movement, and Beresford (2005a) argues that perhaps any negative connotations can be transcended in this context of seeking social change, in much the same way as the notion of disability has been reframed by disability activists. Though we acknowledge the limitations of the term *service user*, it does have currency both in terms of everyday usage within health and social care services, universities and the policy context and it can be seen to have a unifying function across various *disability* and *care* categories to describe:

> . . . *people who receive, have received or are eligible for health and social care services, particularly on a longer term basis* (Beresford, 2005a: 471).

This definition is flexible enough to bring into its compass people, usually in a context of mental health, who prefer the term *survivor*, and those people who though *eligible* for services, for a variety of reasons choose not to access them.

Our book is about the experiences of service users *and* carers. We do not suggest that these groups are coterminous or share experiences and aims; though there is undoubtedly some common ground, there are also some key differences of interests. Rather, this book is about the involvement of service users *and* carers in universities. Throughout the text, we will refer to *service users and carers* where both have a stake in the topic, but will differentiate as necessary between the two groups. On occasion, the term service user may be used as shorthand for *service users and carers*, where it is clear that both sets of stakeholders are involved, if a degree of succinctness is called for and this can be achieved without compromising clarity.

Introduction

The subject matter of this book is the involvement within universities of people with experience of using health and social care services and informal carers. The main focus is how their knowledge and expertise, born out of personal experiences, can be brought to bear in improving the quality of teaching and learning. Our interest does not stop here, however, and associated involvement ranges over research and other activity within higher education institutions, which can take place independently of teaching but, ideally, connects with and supports the pedagogical enterprise. It is also necessary to acknowledge the socio-political context and issues relating to setting, which firmly locate universities as community based institutions. As such, engagement on this territory raises some key points of interest about the civic role of universities and their relationship with their communities.

Structure of the Book

We have divided the text into two broad sections. The respective sections group chapters thematically under the two headings:

1. The context. This section includes Chapter 1 to 5 and offers discussion of key issues in service user and carer involvement and the role of universities with reference to available theoretical accounts and published literature.
2. Personal experiences: the case of Comensus. This section covers Chapters 6 to 9 and engages with practical applications of theory, addressing service user and carer involvement in universities in practice. Real world examples and personal biographical accounts are drawn on, with key material included from our own experiences within the Comensus initiative at the University of Central Lancashire (UCLan).

The book concludes with a short closing chapter that attempts to synthesise material from the two sections, draw some key overarching conclusions, and outline some aspirations for the future.

The *context* section opens with a general chapter on *Service User and Carer Involvement in Higher Education*. This first chapter reviews developments in the field and places these in a context of general policy background. There is clearly a wealth of engagement between universities and health and social care service users and carers, and the numbers of projects are growing apace. The literature is drawn on to explore the degree to which different reported involvement initiatives embody features of authentic collaboration or partnership, with reference to the analytic framework provided by a notion of a *ladder of involvement*. Reflections on a hierarchy of involvement, from negligible involvement and paternalism to complete involvement and partnership, help to identify key enablers and barriers for effective participation.

Chapter 2 explores *The Social and Political Context* and considers the growth of service user and carer involvement in university settings as possibly part of a wider social movement. Literature and theory developed in the study of social movements can be applied to this specific context affording interesting insights into people's motivations to take part, factors that sustain involvement and relationships and connections within and between groups.

Issues pertinent to the location of universities within their local communities are taken up in Chapter 3: *Beyond the Campus: Universities, Community Engagement and Social Enterprise*. This chapter analyses the different ways in which service user and carer interests are served in various community groups and voluntary sector settings in a context of civic and community engagement. Concepts of social capital, social enterprise and social marketing are critically reviewed and reflected upon for their utility in supporting user and carer involvement. The different ways in which universities can connect with this activity, as supporter or beneficiary, are described as a point of departure for consideration of the notion of a critically engaged institution.

Making the case for service user and carer involvement is greatly assisted in university settings by reference to available research findings. The imperative to properly evaluate novel initiatives is reflected in the content of Chapter 4: *Research and Evaluation of Service Users' and Carers' Involvement in Health Professional Education*. This chapter deals with systematic research methods as well as the more routine audit, evaluation and quality assurance of user or carer involvement. The content of this chapter mainly addresses discussion of relevant methodological approaches, with a more detailed account of outcomes being the focus of Chapter 5.

Chapter 5 addresses the topic of *Outcomes*. In order to determine which outcomes matter, the theoretical basis for health and social care is examined. This is contextualised by the positions of the stakeholders who might have an interest in the commissioning, provision and outcomes of health and social care education. A binary model of professional education is described, with two axes, one of clinical competence and knowledge, the other of attitudes and values. Through an exploration of service user engagement as a complex salutogenic endeavour, the chapter hypothesises that one of the primary outcomes of service user and carer engagement might be the development of moral and ethical maturity in care givers, manifest as emotional intelligence. This provides an essential counter-balance to the clinical and knowledge based weighting of professional education that pertains in the absence of such engagement.

Section Two of the book includes some significant contributions from people either directly involved in the UCLan Comensus initiative, or connected to it in some way. The weight given to this case material is, we feel, justified given the unique approach to systematic involvement across a whole Faculty. It is opportune then, at this juncture, to briefly introduce this particular service user and carer involvement programme. The Comensus initiative has been growing since 2004 in the Faculty of Health at UCLan (Downe *et al.*, 2007). It is an attempt to develop a systematic and comprehensive framework of user and carer involvement that extends into all aspects of the Faculty's work: teaching, research and strategic decision making. The name is not quite an acronym, representing a notion of Community Engagement and Service User Involvement in a University with Support.

Comensus has attempted from the outset to tackle some of the challenges posed by a reading of the literature. We were probably not unique in our own particular starting point, wherein there was a critical mass of academics and community participants connected to the university and interested in user and carer involvement, but previous activity had been piecemeal and uncoordinated. Starting with an affinity for participatory approaches to enquiry and development, and with a commitment to the realization of genuine rather than tokenistic ends, we embarked upon a journey of discovery wrapped up in an action research methodology. The different ways in which participants are supported and support each other has come to be a crucial and valued feature of this work. Along the way we have strengthened established relationships and made new ones with service users, carers, community groups and academics affiliated to our university and other higher education institutions, in this country and abroad. In many respects, it is these relationships and connections which have helped the writing of this book.

Chapter 6 describes and reflects upon the challenges in *Setting up Comensus*, told from the point of view of the person responsible for coordinating the initiative. A portion of the chapter deals with wider theories of organizational culture and how this can be changed by service user and carer involvement. Of course, the chapter also deals with some of the impediments or barriers to change in higher education institutions. The importance of all involved sharing key values and principles associated with authentic involvement is highlighted if these barriers are to be overcome.

As a counterpoint to Chapter 6, the material in Chapter 7 points out the importance of institutional leadership and the capacity to influence systems of bureaucracy and management from the inside. *Climbing the Ladder of Involvement: A Manager's Perspective* describes aspects of these processes and one manager's personal journey in relation to institutional progress towards partnership working in practice.

In Chapter 8 a number of biographical *Stories of Engagement* are presented that span service user, carer, academic staff, involvement development worker and collegiate network coordinator perspectives on service user and carer involvement in university settings. These serve to cast light on the richness and diversity of people's experiences, and the extent to which these endeavours attract compliments and criticism.

In Chapter 9 we return to some of the analyses of social movements first encountered in Chapter 2. These themes are illuminated with reference to the actual ways in which service user and carer participants within Comensus talk about their involvement and how they make sense of it for themselves. These narratives have been collected as part of the action research study that shaped the development of the Comensus initiative.

In some respects, Chapter 10 returns to our opening concerns about the importance of language and terminology. In *Shedding Masks: Transitions in Mental Health and Education, a Personal View*, one individual passionately rejects the constraining aspects of the label *service user*. The humanistic writings of Maslow and Freire are cited to inform a discussion of individuality, creativity and expression. This polemic continues to resonate with a desire to make a positive difference for others, but strives to shake off demeaning features of the appellation *service user* towards reclaiming a positive sense of self and personal identity not defined in terms of health status or service usage.

All of the contributors to this text and, we are sure, many of you, the readers of it, have been involved in some way or other with service user and carer contributions to education, research or other activity in universities or wider communities. In all of this work, and in the production of this book, we have all learnt from each other and engaged in positive, productive and even life-affirming relationships. The first things that become apparent in this context are the enthusiasm and commitment of community participants to make a difference in the university and ultimately endeavour to effect real changes to the actual practice and organization of health and social care services. We hope that the pages of this book reflect the wealth of good practice and learning that is evident in the various examples of university, service user and carer partnerships that are to be found, and in some way make a contribution to the aforementioned goals.

Part I: The Context

1 Service User and Carer Involvement in Higher Education

I never thought that I would be involved with a university's teaching and learning – possibly sweeping the floor would have been the only way in.

1.1 Introduction

There has been a general trend over recent decades towards acceptance of the notion that the public ought to have a more participatory role in the state, and that people who make use of various services have a particular interest in decision making and planning as well as the nature of service they receive. This general consumerism has been influential in United Kingdom policy relating to health and social care, and in specific institutions of care delivery (DH, 2005, 2006a; HM Government, 2007). Often coming from a different ideological position, the same ends have been pursued by a burgeoning social movement of service users and community groups. Most recently, the notions of personalisation and personalised care have come to the foreground in analyses of service failings and prescriptions for reform (Carr, 2008). This trend is evident in the Darzi review of the UK National Health Service (NHS) and the growing adoption of individual budgets in the social care field in particular (HM Government, 2007; DH, 2008, 2009a).

The idea that people should have a say in the planning, delivery and evaluation of their care, and that their views should be respected and acted upon by practitioners, is almost taken for granted in the United Kingdom, and in other resource rich countries, such as Canada. A natural extension of this expansion of participation is to create and sustain similar opportunities for involvement in higher education institutions, where health and social care staff are trained, and where relevant academic research staff are located. This has been matched by a global interest in collaborative approaches to interprofessional learning and workforce development that also bring service users and carers in to the partnership and promote community engagement (Hargadon and Staniforth, 2000; Barr *et al.*, 2005; Freeth *et al.*, 2005; Meads *et al.*, 2005; Hammick *et al.*, 2009). Over the last few years, a great deal of interest has developed in methods of developing and supporting such an endeavour. This has resulted in the production of numerous reviews, guidelines and position statements for involvement activity, in service delivery (Crawford *et al.*, 2002; Public Administration Select Committee, 2008), in research (Beresford, 2005b; Hanley, 2005; Involve, 2007), and in education and training (Wykurz and Kelly, 2002; Repper and Breeze, 2007; Tew, Gell and Foster, 2004; Branfield *et al.*, 2007).

A wealth of interesting initiatives has been developed across the range of universities with a stake in the education of health and social care staff and research in the field. These include involvement in all aspects of teaching and learning, such as curriculum planning, lesson planning, delivery of teaching sessions, course and module management, assessment of student progress and wider quality assurance processes (Downe *et al.*, 2007). Service users and carers have also been at the centre of various innovations in practitioner education, such as enquiry or problem-based learning (Dammers, Spencer and Thomas, 2001), e-learning and distance learning (Simpson *et al.*, 2008), and simulated patient sessions (Morris, Armitage and Symonds, 2005; Priestley, Hellawell and McKeown, 2007). This involvement extends into the arena of interprofessional learning and collaboration, which is transacted in both universities and the workplace (Meads *et al.*, 2005). In the United Kingdom, various professional reviews and regulatory bodies who have oversight of curriculum development have advocated both user involvement and interprofessional learning (DH, 2006b; GSCC, 2005).

Involvement in research can be at different stages of the process, but there have been few examples of extensive involvement throughout a research study, or, indeed, of completely user-led research, though this is growing (Lowes and Hulatt, 2005; Pitts and Smith, 2007; Sweeney *et al.*, 2009). In a context of wider community engagement, involvement in participatory action research approaches offers a promising route to more complete engagement, opportunities for authentic user-led research studies and opening up the civic role of higher education institutions (Hanley, 2005; Holdsworth and Quinn, 2006; Church, Shragge, Fontain and Ng, 2008).

The development of service user and carer involvement in universities has been piecemeal. New initiatives have evolved because of the activity of key individuals, rather than always being effectively planned and supported at the institutional level. Reflecting this, resources and funding are a perennial problem for a number of university initiatives and projects, raising real questions about sustainability. There are a few exceptions to the rule. In the United Kingdom, ring-fenced funding is available in relation to social work training and, despite its relatively low level, these monies have been valuable in developments associated with social work. A number of networks have grown up to support people interested in relevant work, for example the Developers of User and Carer Involvement in Education (DUCIE) network hosted by the Mental Health in Higher Education (mhhe) initiative. There have also been a number of international conferences and scholarly meetings focused on health and social care services user and carer involvement in universities, including the foundational *Where's the Patient Voice Conference* (Farrell, Towle and

Godolphin, 2006) and the University of Central Lancashire (UCLan) *Authenticity to Action Conference*.

International efforts to involve service users and carers in higher education settings are too numerous to list. Some examples from different international contexts that have had a systemic impact are noted here. In Australia an alternative approach has been the direct employment of a service user in an academic post, referred to as consumer academic, with the remit of encouraging greater consumer involvement within the Centre of Psychiatric Research, the provision of a consumer perspective and, ultimately, greater acceptance of consumer involvement by academics (Happell, Pinikahana and Roper, 2002). A number of United Kingdom universities have appointed development workers to academic posts to support user and carer involvement. Many of these appointments are of people with personal experience as service users, including notable examples at City University, London, and the University of Leeds, both in the United Kingdom. In Toronto, Canada, well developed relationships between Ryerson University and a range of community groups and individuals have led to a number of interesting collaborative developments. There is *A History of Madness* course open to all students of the university designed and taught by David Reville, mental health service survivor and community activist. In a lengthy partnership, mental health service users and academic staff have worked together to establish and evaluate a range of social businesses using participatory action research approaches (Church, 1997). In the United States, *Community and Physicians Together* is a joint venture between the University of California, Davis, a local health care provider and 10 community organizations in the Sacramento area. Doctors in training are allocated to community groups where people from the community assist in teaching them about their individual health needs and how best to make a difference to health at a community level. This initiative was awarded the Campus Compact Thomas Ehrlich Award for Civically Engaged Faculty in 2008 (Paterniti *et al.*, 2006). The Comensus initiative at UCLan has attempted to develop a systematic approach to user and carer involvement that covers a whole Faculty and reaches other university business and Faculties (Downe *et al.*, 2007). At Brunel University, London, Peter Beresford, mental health service user and activist, has held a chair since 1998 in the Centre for Citizen Participation, and has made a significant contribution to pushing forward issues of user involvement in both education and research in United Kingdom universities.

This book deals with alliances between universities and service users and carers at a number of different levels: people who have experienced significant use of health or social care services, those who care for sick or disabled relatives, those who choose not to use services for various reasons, those who experience stigma or social exclusion linked to a health condition or disability, those who wish to celebrate positive experiences and examples of good practice and those who have had negative experiences and need to address examples of poor practice. All have a stake in the activity of universities. This may be in terms of seeking influence or direct participation in the range of university business, or it may be in attempting to harness the resources of the university to support individuals and groups to tackle concerns arising in the community. The most obvious means of engagement is involvement in the training and education of the health and social care workforce as a vehicle for effecting desired changes in service provision. Similarly, involvement in research activity can be potentially influential in making services better. At a more complex level, closer relationships between community participants and academic staff can begin to subtly or significantly transform working practices in universities and their inter-relationship with the community.

> The primary reason for involving service users in the training and education of mental health professionals is the anticipation that it will produce practitioners capable of delivering improved and more relevant outcomes for users and their carers. (Tew *et al.*, 2004)

This premise has seen a number of universities in a range of countries setting up service user and carer involvement initiatives that strive to incorporate service user and carer perspectives in the education of future generations of practitioners (Barr, 2005; Church, 2005; Church, Bascia and Shragge, 2008). This range of involvement is often linked to wider community engagement activity, with the relationship between universities and their local communities of significant importance to all parties (McNay, 2000; Cone and Payne, 2002; Savan, 2004; Winter, Wiseman and Muirhead, 2006; Campus Compact, 2009). At this level, individuals and community groups will begin to have a strategic voice within universities, addressing key concerns, such as widening access or reciprocal use of resources, or academic knowledge and power may be mobilised to support community campaigns. In such a context, interesting questions arise concerning identity, with academic and lay identities open for transformation or entrenchment (Church, 1996; Spandler and McKeown, 2008).

Arguably, health and social care professionals need to be equipped to involve service users and carers in both personal and strategic decisions. An understanding of relevant social and political factors can be seen as crucial to this enterprise. For this to happen, future health and social care practitioners need to be given the skills as soon as possible within their training and should regard this involvement as standard and not merely as an add on to practice. In seeking full and empowered participation, service user and disability activists rally behind the clarion call of *nothing about us, without us*. This echoes the classic feminist stance, in which the personal is most definitely political.

1.2   The Politics of Health and Welfare

Conventional welfare provision in the United Kingdom has been criticised as paternalistic. This is taken to mean that interventions are carried out for the perceived good of service users by those seen as authoritative experts. Systems built on this premise have led to doctors, social workers and nurses being afforded status and authority, with service users and carers deferring to their specialist knowledge and expertise. At its worst, this approach leads to the service user or carer having minimal input into any care regime, and feelings of disempowerment, confusion and uncertainty occur.

Means and Smith (1998: 71) suggest:

> There is no simple answer as to what does and what does not represent user empowerment, since it is a contested concept. However, most would argue that it involves users taking or being given more power over decisions affecting their welfare.

Change within health and social care services is slow. However, two drivers have been significant in bringing the voice of service users and carers to the fore. These are:

1. The growth of consumerism, latterly associated with a personalization agenda.
2. The growth and status of a number of service user and carer movements campaigning for transformation of services.

In the 1980s and early 1990s public services in the United Kingdom and elsewhere became heavily influenced by the notion of consumerism. Users of services were seen as customers who could exercise choice about the care they received. The development of consumerism in the United Kingdom health and welfare context grew out of a prevailing neo-liberal political ideology strongly associated with the Conservative government of Margaret Thatcher. This New Right philosophy highlighted the need to promote individual choice, roll back the welfare state and expand the influence of the private sector within health and social care. Notwithstanding claims to the contrary, the advent of a New Labour government in 1997 did little to diminish the broad privatization agenda. There has been a progressive critique of these policies, particularly in relation to their lack of adaptability to health and social care. Consumerism has, however, opened up various empowerment strategies for service user and carer movements. It has done this by emphasizing that every individual is a citizen with a set of social, civil and political rights. Users and carers have carried out collective action congruent with this premise and, as a result, changes in legislation, policy and practice have come about. Whilst service user movements have to some extent taken advantage of the political opportunity afforded by the rise of consumerism, movement politics are more complex and, arguably, have much more in common with the progressive left and strands of anarchist political thought than with the new right. Those seeking organizational change within universities come up against various structural and cultural barriers that need to be understood and overcome.

1.3 Organizational Culture and Culture Change

The concept of culture within organizations has been thought of and defined in different, diverse and sometimes contradictory ways. For Geert Hoefstede (2001: 9), culture is *'the collective programming of the mind that distinguishes the members of one group or category of people from another'.* Diana Pheysey (1993: 19) also sees culture in this way, stating that culture is *'a programmed way of seeing derived from beliefs and values'.* Deal and Kennedy (1982) also ally themselves to these theories believing that *'a strong culture is a system of informal rules that spell out how people are to behave most of the time'.* Essentially, *'it is the way we do things around here'.* Robbins (2001) defines organizational culture as the social glue that helps to hold an organization together. Andrew Brown's (1998: 9) definition articulates well the interplay between inculcation of collective values and norms of behaviour in the culture of organizations:

> Organisational culture refers to the patterns of beliefs, values and learned ways of coping with experience that have developed during the course of an organisation's history, and which tend to be manifested in its material arrangements and behaviours of its members.

Peters and Waterman (1982) claim that *'excellent companies are marked by very strong cultures'.* However, this is not necessarily the case. As Brown (1998) notes in his 'consistency hypothesis', strong cultures do not equate with high performance where inconsistency between the espoused culture and culture in practice is present.

> Those who advocate culture management tend to assume that culture is a variable that is easily identified and manipulable. (Woodall, 1996: 27)

Jean Woodall implies that the management of culture is problematic. Brown (1998) agrees with Woodall's perception but states that the difficulties are of a relative rather than an absolute nature and that to manage culture requires *'the ability both to introduce change and to maintain the status quo'* (Brown, 1998: 161). This dichotomy can be evident in universities, where the espoused culture may welcome service user and carer involvement but established hierarchies, bureaucratic systems and processes, entrenched throughout these organizations, ensure that cultural change is difficult to realise. This issue is illustrated in Chapter 6, using the specific example of the Comensus initiative.

Schein's (1985) levers for change advocate that managers should engage in actions in an attempt to manipulate their employees. Such manipulation is often met by resistance to change. Robbins (2001) differentiates between individual and organizational resistance to change. He cites individual sources of resistance as habit, need for security, fear of the unknown, economic factors, selective information processing and myopia. Organizational sources of resistance are structural inertia, limited focus on change, group inertia, threats to expertise, power relationships and established resource allocations. Some of these resistors to change are clearly apparent in universities; where academics are seen as the experts along with associated power imbalances.

Some universities have strong cultures and emphasise a clear mission. Whilst some authors celebrate strong cultures (Peters and Waterman, 1982) believing them to be a recipe for success, others argue that strong organizational cultures can be oppressive and reduce innovation, making change difficult to accomplish (Flynn and Chatman, 2001).

> The stronger the culture, the harder it is to change. Culture causes organisational inertia; it is the brake that resists change because this is precisely what culture should do – protect the organisation from willy-nilly responses to fads and short term fluctuations. (Deal and Kennedy, 1982: 159)

Ogbonna (1992: 8) agrees with this stance and argues that 'the ability to manage culture implies not just a capacity to change and maintain it, but to create, abandon and destroy it as well'.

Adoption into core areas of performance may be a route to more profound organizational cultural change. As Pennington (2003: 251) states:

> The truth is that culture change is driven by a change in performance. An organisation's culture cannot be installed. It can be guided and influenced by the policies, practices, skills and procedures that are implemented and reinforced. The only way to change the culture is to change the way individuals perform on a daily basis.

For this change to happen, Pennington suggests five basic ideas for performance change: create a business related sense of urgency; focus on performance by setting specific goals, and measure everything; change systems and structures in addition to skills; make change a way of life; and, finally, create opportunities for ownership.

There is a risk that these approaches may result in enforced change that is not fully embedded in the values of organizational members. Despite the widespread acceptance of the validity of service user and carer involvement, it is possible that complex higher education organizations defy easy systematic integration of such involvement. Possible reasons for this might be the differing value base of stakeholders. Career bureaucrats, academics and lay participants may all have a commitment to increased user and carer involvement for entirely different reasons. In the university context, the various health and social care practice disciplines may also exhibit historically entrenched features of professional identity and socialization, associated with enduring claims to power that can operate to limit the realization of transformative goals (Luke, 2003). Significant cultural change can, possibly, only occur within the organization if all parties are authentically attached to altruistic and equity based values which would define a truly service user and carer led initiative.

1.4 Policy and Implementation

In the United Kingdom context, the agenda of authentically involving service users and carers in the development, delivery and evaluation of professional education in health and social care is gaining importance within services (DH, 1994a,

1998a, 2000a, 2001a, 2004a; NHS Executive, 1999) and with professional bodies such as the General Medical Council (GMC, 1993) and the General Social Care Council (GSCC/SCIE, 2004). This involvement has grown in prominence due to a combination of legislation and the recognition by professional bodies that, if future health and social care practitioners are to be prepared to work in user-led services (DH, 2005), then there is a need for their input within all spheres of training, from the clinical practice arena to the classroom.

> Curriculum developers should recognise the important role of carers and users in advising on service provision and development. Consultation processes should be wide ranging and representatives of service users and carers should be involved where practicable in the development, delivery and evaluation of curriculum. (National Board for Nursing and Midwifery for Scotland, 2000: 4)

Involving service users and carers in the education of future health and social care practitioners provides students with a unique insight into lived experience, grounds education in reality, enhances the students' experience, provides an added dimension to teaching and empowers the service user and carer. Few universities have responded comprehensively to the call for involvement, and critics suggest that involvement in practitioner education has been inconsistent (Basset, 1999). This highlights the need to examine current initiatives and examine the scope, remit and effectiveness of such activity.

Health and social care policy requires service user and carer involvement in practice, research and education, but evidence of its impact, scope and the influence of such involvement need to be investigated. There is a growing body of literature surrounding service user and carer involvement in education and research in universities and wider community engagement (Repper and Breeze, 2007). The main focus has arguably been on literature documenting the experience of higher education institutions (HEIs) and their attempts to involve service users and carers in their scholarly activities, their successes and any barriers they have faced.

1.5   Representation

The vexed issue of representation and representativeness is a key focus of debate amongst interested parties, typified by challenges of contested meaning, and can be a potential avenue for service agencies or institutions to devalue or embargo the input of particular individuals or groups (Beresford and Campbell, 1994). Concerns around representation include issues such as how people can speak for others or from a general perspective, perceived credibility and validity around who is involved and questions over why these individuals are representative of the wider service user/carer populace. The British Psychological Society (2008: 18) discussed this notion within its 'Good Practice Guidelines' and decided that 'representativeness should be an aspiration not an obstacle'. This notion is also discussed widely by Robert *et al.* (2003: 63):

Professionals wishing to promote user involvement frequently express concerns about the representativeness of individual service users, sometimes suggesting that particular service users may be 'too well', 'too articulate' or too vocal to represent the views of users more general'.

Crawford (2001: 85) responds to this criticism by pointing out that 'this problem is not specific to those representing the views of service users. The same question could be asked of those representing the views of local general practitioners, psychiatrists etc.'

We would recommend that we accept un-representativeness as each person who has experienced services/or cared for someone who has experienced services has a unique insight and contribution to make.

Practical methods to combat this issue within education have been suggested by City University in its guidelines for 'User and Carer Involvement in Educational Activity'. These include:

- Users and carers nominating representatives themselves from their groups.
- The fostering of local relationships.
- Transparency and flexibility.
- Always involving more than one service user or carer.

1.6   Level of Involvement

Even though the agenda of involving service users and carers in the education of future health and social care practitioners is gaining in importance, achieving meaningful involvement is complex, defying simple remedies. The extent to which involvement is authentic and meaningful for participants is crucial, and a number of commentators have attempted to represent progressive stages towards more complete involvement. Arnstein (1969) introduced the concept of movement across a continuum of participation. Arnstein's 'ladder of citizen participation' includes (in descending order of power) – sharing, citizen control, delegated power, partnership, placation, consultation, informing, therapy and manipulation.

Tew, Gell and Foster (2004) developed this model of a continuum further in their 'ladder of involvement' and related it directly to mental health education (Table 1.1):

The premise is that for any initiative in which service users or carers are involved development will occur, hopefully advancing up the ladder. For instance, the process will move service users and carers from being passive recipients to fully engaged, equal partners in education. According to the scope and range of their involvement, different initiatives can be placed at different levels on the ladder. The literature describes a number of schemes that, whilst attempting full partnership, fall short of reaching this ideal. Typically, these initiatives tend to focus on classroom participation.

Table 1.1   Ladder of Involvement (Tew, Gell and Foster, 2004: 54)

Level 1 No involvement	The curriculum is planned, delivered and managed with no consultation or involvement of service users or carers
Level 2 Limited involvement	Outreach and liaison with local service user and carer groups. Service users/carers invited to 'tell their story' in a designated slot, and/or be consulted ('when invited') in relation to course planning or management, student selection, student assessment or programme evaluation. Payment offered for their time. No opportunity in shaping the course as a whole
Level 3 Growing involvement	Service users/carers contributing regularly to at least two of the following in relation to a course or module: planning, delivery, student selection, assessment, management or evaluation. Payment for teaching activities at normal lecturer rates. However, key decisions on matters such as curriculum content, learning outcomes or student selection may be made in forums in which service users/carers are not represented. Some support available to contributors before and after sessions, but no consistent programme of training and supervision offered. No discrimination against service users and carers accessing programmes as students.
Level 4 Collaboration	Service users/carers are involved as full team members in at least three of the following in relation to a course or module: planning, delivery, student selection, assessment, management or evaluation. This is underpinned by a statement of values and aspirations. Payment for teaching activities at normal visiting lecturer rates. Service users/carers contributing to key decisions on matters such as curriculum content, style of delivery, learning outcomes, assessment criteria and methods, student selection and evaluation criteria. Facility for service users/ carers who are contributing to the programme to meet up together, and regular provision of training, supervision and support. Positive steps to encourage service users and carers to access programmes as students.
Level 5 Partnership	Service users, carers and teaching staff work together systematically and strategically across all areas – and this is underpinned by an explicit statement of partnership values. All key decisions made jointly. Service users and carers involved in the assessment of practice learning. Infrastructure funded and in place to provide induction, support and training to service users and carers. Service users and carers employed as lecturers on secure contracts, or long-term contracts established between programmes and independent service user or carer training groups. Positive steps made to encourage service users and carers to join in as participants in learning sessions even if they are not (yet) in a position to achieve qualifications.

1.7   Models and Approaches

1.7.1   Limited Involvement – The Ladder of Involvement Level 2

Service users and carers are frequently invited into universities to talk of their experiences of using health and social services in a dedicated teaching session. This is by no means a new phenomenon:

For the junior student in medicine and surgery it is a safe rule to have no teaching without a patient for a text, and the best teaching is that taught by the patient himself. (William Osler, 1905 quoted in Spencer *et al.*, 2000: 851)

Involving service users and carers in this way allows the student to listen to and recognise the unique experience of health and social care that people have had. It also brings to the fore the influence that social inequalities and stigma have on patients lives. The recognition of the persons' own definition of their experiences can be seen as both empowering and validating (Campbell and Lindow, 1997).

Wood and Wilson Barnett (1999) set up a small research project to include mental health service users in classroom work. The outcomes from the research indicated that those students who had experienced service users and carers in the classroom were less likely to use jargon, more able to empathise, and more likely to view service users as individuals, and not patients with medical labels. In a report on the development of a course for cancer nurses, Flanagan (1999) recognised that user involvement in the classroom leads to greater empathy. This is borne out by Spencer *et al.* (2000) who stress that direct student-service user contact can enhance a student's ability to understand the actual experience of ill health.

Costello and Horne (2001) carried out an evaluative study involving the use of patients in the classroom. One student stated, 'It was beneficial to listen to a patient telling you about actual experiences rather than a teacher telling you about hypothetical ones'. Another reported, 'You received answers that you would not find in a text book'. From the data, 56% of the respondents indicated that a great deal had been learnt from the session, and 85% of the respondents agreed that the involvement of service users helped them to gain a greater understanding of their problems.

Despite the undoubted enthusiasm amongst students in this study to hear first hand of the service users' experiences, this involvement could be deemed as tokenistic. When mapped against the 'Ladder of Involvement' it would be characterised as limited (Level 2). Beresford and colleagues (2006: 327) speak of the dangers of tokenism within social work education:

On many social work courses the most that might happen could be one session led by service users, often with little support from the college, when they were encouraged to talk about themselves and their problems rather than their views and ideas about what social workers should be doing.

While low levels of involvement can be criticised as tokenistic, the research undertaken by Khoo and colleagues (2004) on the impact service users have on Masters students' educational experiences found evidence that reasonably simple involvement of service users in a classroom setting can pose effective learning challenges for students. The study was carried out in two phases. In phase one, a short questionnaire was sent out to students. In phase two, a sample of ten respondents was interviewed. From the questionnaire 79% of respondents rated the contribution of service users as good to excellent. Collectively, user involvement was found to convey a number of benefits for course participants. Students reported that the service user sessions:

- Helped ground practice in reality.
- Raised awareness of issues and of user perspectives.
- Provided a focus on partnership.
- Challenged existing approaches.
- Challenged participants' personal views of the world.
- Raised participants' confidence as practitioners.
- Enabled informed change.

Some of these observations suggest the transformational potential of service user involvement in the classroom, beyond the sort of tokenism highlighted by authors such as Beresford. It follows from Beresford and colleagues' (2006) commentary that the meaningfulness of this involvement depends upon adequate planning and support, elements that are also amenable to a participatory approach.

Scheyett and Diehl (2006: 436) recognise the incongruity between the ethos of partnership in professional practice and the role of partnership in social work education:

> Social work educators, if we are to act in congruence with our values, must examine the extent to which we practice partnership, self determination and empowerment in our curriculum development and in the educational process itself.

1.7.2   Growing Involvement and Collaboration – The Ladder of Involvement Levels 3 and 4

Involvement which goes beyond occasional teaching sessions is happening within some education establishments. Flanagan (1999) engaged users and carers in the design of continuing and higher education in cancer care nursing within the University of Leeds School of Healthcare Studies. The design team met over a number of months within course design meetings, and *'the lessons from this particular example of public involvement were positive for all parties'* (Flanagan, 1999). The study goes on to conclude that, for all the good intentions of professionals, there is no substitute for the direct involvement of service users and carers. These valuable insights and perceptions were seen to be essential in the education of future cancer nurse specialists.

Dammers, Spencer and Thomas (2001) used real people in problem-based learning. 69 students over a two-year period studied a problem-based learning module attached to the undergraduate medical curriculum at Newcastle University Medical School. All completed a questionnaire. In response to the question, 'Was there any particular added value in having real as opposed to paper cases for the problems?', all the students expressed positive value in having service user involvement. The Newcastle team conclude that the use of active participants in problem-based learning should be considered more widely.

Arguably, including service users and carers in education should be a true partnership with engagement across all aspects of the curriculum. Authors have identified that there is a need for both organizational and individual commitment if the inclusion of users and carers as experts is to be more than a token gesture or a sop to political rhetoric. Tew and colleagues (2004: 57) point out that:

> ...achieving effective service user and carer involvement involves a significant commitment of time, along with relationship building, strategic planning and problem solving skills; all of this needs to be underpinned by appropriate funding and an infrastructure for support.

The Open University (OU) came to similar conclusions, and went further by exploring power imbalances in a narrative describing the production of a mental health course. The Open University designated resources, including time and money, for service user involvement in the production of an Open University course on mental health. This involvement provided educators with many dilemmas, as they had to work to fulfil academic criteria whilst balancing this against sensitivity and respect for service user perspectives. Jim Read, a notable movement activist wrote about this process:

> Decision-making was all too often based on money and power, rather than sensitivity towards the people who would most be affected. It also stirred up my concerns about working with academics, who I perceived as potentially over-concerned with a false notion of balance as opposed to listening to the voices of oppressed people. (Reynolds and Read, 1999: 423)

The course team had differing views as to the extent and format of service user contributions. Service user members of the group commented that to include service users and not take on board what is said was tokenism. Service users became angry and the situation became stressful. Over time, with negotiation, compromise was reached. The course team commented that they learnt to be more sensitive to power relationships and to be clear about the decision making process.

Simons and colleagues (2007) took a slightly different approach to inclusion and carried out an observational study to evaluate the development of a Service User Academic Post and its impact in terms of social inclusion. A service user was employed by the university to take the involvement agenda forward. This post would have the same status, terms and conditions as for any other educator, although the job title was unique. The findings from the study indicated that, although the post was intended to be integrated into the teaching team, the post holder was not actually involved in 'normal educator activities'. This singled the post holder out as being different. On the positive side, fellow academics pointed to the symbolic power of the existence of the post in the institution. They remarked that appointing a service user moved the institution 'beyond rhetoric to action', and demonstrated that the academic team were willing to 'put our money where our mouth is'. The importance of building relationships in the team was also stressed:

> The user academic would make sure there were user/carer strands through everything. She was good at that because she did actually form good working relationships with most

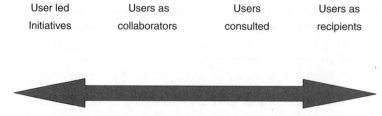

User led	Users as	Users	Users as
Initiatives	collaborators	consulted	recipients

Figure 1.1 Continuum of participation – services and education. Reproduced from Lathlean *et al.* (2006: 734) with kind permission of Elsevier.

of the team. So she was able to say, 'Where is the user/carer bit in that, then?'. (Educator 2, in Simons *et al.*, 2007)

The findings from this study recognised that user involvement had a positive effect on student learning and that the user academic also had a positive impact on the academic team.

A very similar project has been developed by the University of Melbourne, which employed what it called a Consumer (Service User) Academic into the Centre for Psychiatric Nursing Research and Practice. Melbourne believed that the involvement of a consumer academic would change the culture and ethos of the taught courses. A questionnaire was distributed to 25 post-graduate nursing students to assess the impact of the post. Findings were typically positive.

The majority of the students endorsed the concept of 'consumer academic' involvement in psychiatric nursing academia. This finding may be particularly significant in terms of accepting new teaching approaches to mental health nursing. (Happell, Pinikahana and Roper, 2002: 248)

Lathlean and colleagues (2006) reported on three initiatives that were reviewed within a symposium and which had the linking feature of moving across a continuum of participation. This continuum moves along a horizontal plane from the right hand side, where users are passive, to the left hand side, which promotes consumer-led initiatives (Figure 1.1).

One of the three initiatives reflected upon was Happell's Consumer Academic post previously reviewed. Lathlean and colleagues viewed this method on their continuum as involving a service user as a collaborator in the delivery of education.

This symposium also reviewed an initiative which has developed a strategy for the inclusion of an external user and carer reference group. Members of the group negotiated the strategy for involvement, which included curriculum advice, planning and delivery of curricula at pre and post registration stages, and review of research proposals. Lathlean and colleagues viewed this approach as being located towards the left hand, more progressive, wing of the continuum, where users are collaborators rather than passive recipients. The final approach considered at the symposium was a study focusing on the participation of mental health service users in the clinical practice decisions of mental health student nurses undertaking their nurse training. This study focused on three key concepts: anti-oppressive practice; contact theory, which proposes increased contact with groups of people leads to more positive attitudes; and moral development.

> The outcomes of the inquiry have been to identify, from a service user and student perspective, professional values which respect the individuality of the person; behaviours and actions which share power and reflect belief in individual potential; and cultural aspects within organisations which enable shared learning and full participation in decision-making. (Lathlean *et al.*, 2006: 736)

This programme has been rated by Lathlean as 'users as collaborators' on the involvement continuum. However, with reference to the 'ladder of involvement', the initiative might best be categorised in the 'growing involvement' stage, as there is no clear support programme in place.

Despite the many excellent examples of service users and carers being involved in universities, many of which are featured elsewhere in this book, a review of the relevant literature has been unable to identify any research papers reporting on initiatives that fit Tew and colleagues' Level 5 Partnership Stage. To explain this anomaly, the next section turns to evidence in the literature that has identified barriers to full involvement.

1.8 Barriers to Involvement

There are a number of barriers to authentic service user and carer involvement in education. These were recognised at a United Kingdom workshop held in Derby in June 2003[1], and reviewed in Basset and colleagues' (2006) seminal paper *Service User/Survivor Involvement in Mental Health Training and Education: Overcoming the Barriers*. Within this paper 10 specific barriers to authentic involvement are identified:

1.8.1 Hierarchies that Exclude

Basset and colleagues identify the hierarchical nature of higher education institutions with built in 'pecking orders,' where only authoritative forms of expertise are valued. Lecturers and academics are deemed as the experts. The inclusion of service users and carers challenges these notions of expertise, and may risk the loss of some authoritative power for some individuals or groups.

> The notion of service users as teachers challenges the perceptions of the role of mental health lecturers as the experts. (Felton and Stickley, 2004: 91)

---

[1] In a similar vein a workshop held in Nottingham in 2005 brought together key development workers for service user and carer involvement. This meeting also identified various impediments to involvement (Chapter 8)

Felton and Stickley cite the work of Paolo Freire (1971) in examining the nature of power in the culture of pedagogy. Arguably, whether it is recognised by academics or not, the maintenance of power is important for teachers in order to maintain status as a dominant group. This has significant implications for the involvement of service users in education in terms of the threat they may represent. Basset (1999) takes up the tokenism charge again, in arguing that much service user and carer involvement is based on appropriation rather than partnership, as power structures remain unchanged.

It would seem that higher education institutions may be culturally resistant to a challenge to their power base. In order to move beyond tokenistic responses to the consumerist challenge, service user involvement requires a change in structure that can only be realised or sustained by those who have power, and who are prepared to share it, or even to let it go altogether.

1.8.2   Stigma and Discrimination

Universities are not free from the forces of discrimination. Service users may be seen as ill people who need 'looking after'. This view does not support equal power relationships, but rather fosters paternalistic approaches. The predominant medical model of some disciplines and the professional mores learnt earlier in academic careers might reinforce this.

As noted above, the project undertaken by Simons and colleagues (2007) identified some problems with stigma and discrimination. The title of 'User Academic' labelled the worker and stigmatised the role, which was in direct contrast to the aims of integrating and valuing people equally. The User Academic was not integrated into everyday normal educator activities. This also led to unintended discriminatory behaviours. Some questions as to whether special employment practices were required for the post holder as a vulnerable service user were raised. However, usual systems for staff were bypassed.

The use of mental health service users in higher education by some academics can be resisted because of discrimination and stigma.

> All the lecturers saw a potential difficulty with the capability of service users in the classroom. For some this included the unpredictability of individuals with mental health problems and their possible inability to cope with the demands of working in education. (Felton and Stickley, 2004: 95)

An uncritical acceptance of this belief reinforces the process of excluding service users from education.

1.8.3   Validation and Accreditation Processes

For Basset and colleagues (2006), validation and accreditation processes usually involve sets of meetings where point-scoring and bullying are not uncommon, and free deployment of jargon and acronyms are the order of the day. They note that, when service users or carers are invited into these forums, the academic culture prevalent in the running of the meetings, and the inaccessibility of the format, often precludes participants from contributing in a meaningful or authentic way.

Despite the rhetorical support for user and carer involvement, active participation cannot take place without support mechanisms that appropriately prepare service users and carers. Indeed, properly empowered participation could lead to modifications to university processes and meetings so that they become more inclusive and user friendly for all those attending. This would, of necessity, involve changes to the behaviour and communication styles of many participating academics. Fiona O'Neill (2002) recognised this, stating that *'it is unlikely that active involvement can take place without appropriate preparation of both professionals and users'*. She goes on to say that *'apart from the capacity building aspect of training activities, joint training of lay representatives and professionals provide a way of facilitating partnership working and learning from each other'*.

1.8.4   Academic Jargon and Put-Downs

Educators, researchers, health and social care professionals are notorious for using academic jargon and professional terminology. This can lead to service users and carers feeling stupid, excluded and unable to fully participate in involvement opportunities. Basset and colleagues (2006) suggest that, to be successful, institutional staff need to speak the language of service users and carers. In support of this, Susie Green (2007) comments that service users should not be plunged into the murky unfathomable rhetoric of organizational and health service jargon. The solution is to recognise and accommodate the fact that there are different, but equally valid, cultures and ways of learning and understanding.

1.8.5   Clever People/Clever Excuses

Basset and colleagues further believe there are many excuses for not including service users and carers. People who work in higher education erect their own barriers to inclusion. Excuses such as *'they will feel out of their depth'*, *'we don't want people to feel they have let us down'*, *'there is not enough time to include people'* and *'they are not representative of our clients'* come up often. This passive resistance to inclusion is just as damaging as direct resistance, in that it creates a subtle undermining of the inclusion agenda.

Felton and Stickley's (2004) research also cited fixation on a notion of representativeness as a barrier to involvement, with four of their participants thinking that service users should be representative for user involvement to be valid. This notion is based on the rationale that individuals should be representative of users of the service as a whole to be able to give a valid user perspective. In response, Crepaz-Keay, Binns and Wilson (1997) point out that by being involved and immersed in educational culture, these users cannot be representative in this sense of the word, as the majority of service users do not have this level of involvement experience. As Tritter and colleagues (2004: 23) note:

> Users, like professionals, will provide input based on their own experience. Being too concerned that involved users are representative, or that all possible users are involved, can get in the way of ensuring that users' views are being used to shape services.

1.8.6   Classifying Knowledge

Basset and colleagues also discuss how the academic world is focused on knowledge, evidence and rigour. Service user and carer involvement is not delivered in this way. Input is experiential, often coming from the heart, aiming for shared emotional connections that will enable change in practice. Teaching is also often aimed at a certain level with pre-set conditions attached. Involving service users and carers enables them to contribute in a way that is unique and individual. This is the very point of the exercise. It is not necessarily amenable to definition at level 2 or 3 of a degree programme. Arguably, it has as its strength the power to move students emotionally, enabling them to reflect on their knowledge and practice no matter what level their academic programme.

> It is only through the use of patient experience knowledge, where patients are enabled to share their illness experiences with health-care professionals, either in practice or through educational processes, that theoretical knowledge firmly grounded on practice knowledge becomes the basis for effective nursing practice. (Warne and McAndrew, 2007: 228)

1.8.7   Individual, not a Team Approach

The desirability of achieving a better trained practitioner workforce more in tune with progressive principles of team working because they have studied and trained together is a key element of worldwide social care and health service modernization policy agendas (WHO, 1987; Hargadon and Staniforth, 2000). Despite this, many of today's higher education institutes are split into schools and departments, creating structural impediments for teaching and learning to cross the boundaries of different professional groupings. Basset and colleagues highlight how this can cause difficulties for service users and carers who may want to contribute widely. Cooper, Braye and Geyer (2004) identified such difficulties with interprofessional education at both pre and post registration levels. Although interprofessional learning is a key component for pre registration social work and nursing education and, in some cases, medical education, there can be problems fitting it easily into the established academic worlds where systems, resources and practice have arguably been set up to meet the needs of different professional bodies. Conversely, where efforts are taken to overcome such barriers, interprofessional learning can be successfully implemented and becomes a vehicle for addressing other partnerships, including the involvement of service users and carers (Meads *et al.*, 2005; Barr *et al.*, 2005). Indeed, with reference to the aforementioned study of interprofessional learning, Cooper and Spencer-Dawe (2006) report improved learning outcomes when service users contributed to teaching compared with practitioners alone. Benefits for involving service users included understanding links between personal experiences and theoretical material, a better appreciation of team working principles and the need to locate service users at the centre of care.

1.8.8 Gaining Access in the First Place

Basset and colleagues' paper points out that individual academics may not know how to access service users and carers who wish to get involved. Conversely, service users and carers may not know how to get involved within higher education. This can lead to the few that do manage to become engaged being over-used, becoming burnt out and, ultimately, being disregarded as 'the usual suspects'. This can severely limit the range of service user voices heard.

The Fran Branfield and Shaping Our Lives (2007) report on user involvement in social work education speaks of how service users can internalise negative assumptions about what they can and cannot achieve. *'Some service users lack the confidence to believe they can participate. For some people it is a huge mountain to climb'.* Gina Tyler (2006) reports on her personal experiences of how some workers offer inauthentic gestures to involve people: *'Involving service users in a tokenistic way achieves nothing other than ticking boxes and fabricating figures, which are then used to measure counterfeit involvement'.*

1.8.9 Bureaucratic Payment Systems

Universities often have finance departments incapable of paying service users and carers on the day, in cash, and in a way that will not affect any benefits they may be claiming. The bureaucracy and audit trail needed to claim items such as travel expenses can preclude some service users and carers who may need reimbursement for outlaid expenses as quickly as possible. Turner and Beresford (2005) found that service users and carers who claim benefits are unclear as to which payments and how much they can be paid, worry about receiving payment, find it difficult to gain appropriate advice, worry about paying taxes, worry they will lose their benefits and find negotiating the rules of payment too daunting to take part in involvement opportunities.

1.8.10 Lack of Support for Trainers/Educators

Bennett and colleagues highlight the need for support, including briefing, debriefing, resources and information. Unfortunately, such support is often not available, leaving the service user vulnerable and often having to deal with emotional distress after reliving what are sometimes traumatic life experiences.

Beresford (2005b) believes two essentials need to be in place for successful service user involvement: access and support. Access includes structured ways to get involved and to get your voice heard. Support is whatever is needed to make the process comfortable. O'Neill (2002), Tew, Gell and Foster (2004), Simpson and Benn (2007), Tyler (2006), Stevens and Tanner (2006), Tew and Hendry (2003), Miller and Walters (2006) and a number of other authors all recommend support is given to service users and carers to ensure that they are prepared, feel confident, gain new skills and become empowered as part of the process of involvement. A supportive infrastructure is also seen as necessary to ensure that getting involved within a university does not unduly put service users and carers under pressure or stress.

1.9   Innovation in Teaching and Learning: An Example

One means of addressing barriers to involvement is in the deployment of innovative teaching and learning technologies. There is relatively little published work specifically focused upon user involvement in e-learning, but one clear example is Simpson and colleagues' work around supporting enquiry-based learning with a user-led e-discussion group at City University (Simpson *et al.*, 2008; Simpson and Reynolds, 2008). Here, Alan Simpson describes how their particular approach to involvement in e-learning was developed and observes how it was received by participating students and service users:

It is always a challenge trying to come up with ways to get mental health nursing students to think about what it is like to be a mental health service user. How do you get them to try and understand what it is like to have a mental health problem or to be admitted to a psychiatric hospital? And, more importantly, how do you get those students to reflect on their own attitudes and behaviour and encourage them to have positive, constructive relationships with service users?

Increasingly, service users are being invited to take part in the education and training of healthcare students and staff in a variety of ways (Simpson, 2006), but we were very excited when we had the idea of getting our students to communicate online with people who had personal experience of mental health problems and services.

We knew a lot of people, including service users, used online discussion and message boards to discuss things, but could we make it work as part of an educational project? As far as we could find out, this had not been tried before, so we couldn't nick anyone else's ideas.

A small group of us, including Ian Light – a service user lecturer who sadly died following the completion of the study – created a secure project site complete with sample discussion threads on the University's web site and put together some publicity materials before making contact with local user groups.

After giving presentations at three mental health day centres, we recruited 12 service users keen to take part. About half of them already used the internet, the others were new to computers and e-mails but training, support and payment were all part of the deal. Around the same time we invited a group of 34 second year mental health nursing students to take part in the project and all agreed.

As we intended to evaluate the study (Simpson *et al.*, 2008), everyone was given written information and provided written consent to take part. Information about the number of e-mail messages read and sent was automatically recorded and 10 of the 12 participants (83%) and 13 of the 34 (38%) students, selected to reflect the range of students, were interviewed by an independent researcher.

Once everyone had been trained and knew how to use the discussion forum, the students sent e-mail questions to the service users on six topics linked to a scenario they had been given. They were encouraged to respond to the questions and it was hoped that spontaneous discussions would develop between and amongst the participants. The students also had to use traditional library resources to research their subjects.

All contributions were monitored by the project team, who very occasionally intervened mainly to encourage participation. After six weeks, the service users were invited to attend presentations by the students on what they had learnt.

The project was an overall success with all students and service users interviewed overwhelmingly positive about the online discussion forum. They valued the discussions, would happily take part in a similar project again and would recommend it to others. They supported increased use of online discussions in healthcare education and had suggestions for topics that could be covered.

Students described the contributions of the service users as 'responsive', 'brilliant', 'excellent', 'fantastic' and 'effective'. Their learning had clearly been influenced to some extent in that four of the six groups of students drew on the discussions in their presentations, with two groups focusing their work on the online interactions. They found that the online forum gave them an insight into personal experiences, improved their communication skills and provided motivation to work on psychiatric wards.

Above all they had acquired an understanding of the service users' experiences of admission to hospital and about the feelings aroused by being spoken to or interacted with in a particular way.

> I think just an idea of, just an impression of how it is to be on a psychiatric ward, that is mainly what kind of things I asked about . . . how they found the atmosphere. What were their fears and what they found to be. . . the most worrying aspects of being in hospital? (Student)

Others identified hearing first hand experiences of the impact of mental illness and distress and reflected on how this could influence their clinical practice.

> I have learnt that maybe in future when I go on my placements, to put some of the things I have learnt on board . . . communication skills or during admission. . . that kind of a thing, so these are the kind of things I have learnt and I try as much as possible to implement in practice and improve more. (Student)

Over half the students (58.8%) logged on and read messages from service users and fellow students. However, it became clear that there was a 'visible' group of 15 (44%) contributing to discussions, with 14 (41%) playing no active part online, despite using the technology during the practice weeks. The tendency not to post e-mails reflects the common experience of any online discussion forum, where 'passive' membership ('lurking') often outweighs active participation, but it also reflected concerns expressed during the study that students lacked confidence in communication.

In contrast, the majority of the service users played an active role online. On average they sent more messages than the students and were more confident in using computer technology than most students. They were keen to take a leading role in the online community and valued contributing to the education of future nurses and of challenging stereotypical and stigmatising views of people with mental health problems. They also learnt things themselves from taking part in the discussions.

The service users were generally positive about the input of the students and thought they asked some good questions, but would have appreciated more discussion on a range of other topics. Others expressed frustration with the limited way in which students asked questions and failed to follow-up responses, although they also cited positive examples.

> But then you had some who were really good, like the one about being admitted onto an acute ward and your experiences and I said about mine and someone wrote saying well how could it have been better, what would you have liked to have happened, which I thought was really positive. (Service User)

There was an awareness that some of the students were hesitant about probing too far, which had led some service users to offer encouragement.

> I know there was one or two students that felt they were not confident enough to ask us, or they did not want to cause us any offence and we e-mailed back, don't worry about it cos like we have had worse. . . I can understand where they were coming from but I think we are made of tougher stuff than that, yeah? (Service User)

Service users spoke of gaining confidence in using computers. Being valued and taken seriously was in itself rewarding and empowering, but above all was a hope that they might be contributing towards positive change in the attitudes of staff and the delivery of mental health services.

Some of the discussions were very emotive for the participants but they were able to positively reframe their survival of difficult life experiences. Several explained how they had benefited from talking about their experiences online as the distance and anonymity afforded by the forum was an advantage, perhaps suggesting the supportive potential of online communities.

The use of an online discussion forum involving mental health service users and students is both possible and highly desirable. Online interactions enabled users to discuss their previous experiences, explain the impact of their care and treatment and encouraged students to consider and reflect on the implications for their own practice.

There is considerable scope to develop similar initiatives across health and social care education and it is clear that service users could and should be at the forefront of that development. Future joint projects between service users and educational researchers might attempt to analyse the impact of online discussions on attitudes and healthcare behaviours in the workplace, because that, of course, is where it really matters. The Bradton virtual community e-learning resource being developed by colleagues at the University of Bradford and University of Central Lancashire, United Kingdom, has relied upon service users and carers as peer researchers and developers to produce a range of video stories, grounded in personal experiences of health and social care services. Participants in this initiative report some misgivings that the electronic resource does not promise to replace opportunities for face-to-face contributions to teaching and learning. Conversely, they can also see the value of so-called re-usable learning objects. For some individuals, their physical or emotional condition is such that delivering lengthy teaching sessions or revisiting material for multiple student groups might prove exhausting. The video material is a useful alternative, as it can supplement or even replace direct teaching sessions. Others with life limiting conditions have spoken movingly of the possibility of legacy effects, where their contribution to student learning lasts beyond their death.

1.10   Conclusion

The involvement of health and social care service users and carers in teaching and research endeavours within universities has become much more prominent. The notion of hierarchies of participation, as presented in the various ladders of involvement deployed for evaluation purposes, reflects an acute concern on the part of participants themselves and key academic staff that particular initiatives evidence 'true', 'genuine' or 'authentic' involvement. Aspirations for partnerships are backed up by numerous examples of best practice guidelines and a critical literature, often authored by service users, focused on how best to shape and support new working.

Honest reflection reveals that most involvement activity falls short of full partnership working, and there are few examples of completely user-led projects. These observations confirm the fact that various institutional and cultural factors can act as barriers to the adoption of best practice, but there is sufficient knowledge now about the existence and operation of these impediments for willing participants to take steps to overcome them or minimise adverse effects. Wider sociopolitical and structural factors are also of interest in considering the potential for success, and it is these issues that are turned to in Chapter 2.

2 The Social and Political Context

Cultures and attitudes are changed by human commonality.

2.1 Introduction

This chapter attempts to locate university involvement in its social and political context, with a particular emphasis on consideration of the possible connections between such initiatives and the broader notion of a service user movement. As discussed in the previous chapter, the rhetoric of involvement and participation for the public at large and, specifically, for service users and carers, is now commonplace within health and social welfare services in many countries. In the United Kingdom it is promoted across systems of policy formulation, care administration, governance and research, with an emphasis on individualised processes of care delivery (DH, 2006a). This has been mirrored in the adoption of similar moves towards greater participation in higher education institutions concerned with the teaching and training of health and social care practitioners, and associated scholarly activity (DH, 2002a; Levin, 2004; Basset, Campbell and Campbell, 2006). Such developments are often nested within a wider rhetorical commitment to community engagement and to advancing the role of the university as a civic body (McNay, 2000; Cone and Payne, 2002; Savan, 2004; Winter, Wiseman and Muirhead, 2006; Campus Compact, 2009).

Service user and carer involvement in higher education has a number of things to commend it, including notable contributions to increased access, wider democratic involvement, supportive mechanisms, debate and an emphasis on collaboration between professionals and 'experts by experience'. Notwithstanding these perceived benefits, the relationship between universities, academic staff, individual service users and carers, and self-organised groups can sometimes be problematic. It can be acutely threatened by fundamental issues, such as entrenchment of stigma, and differentials in status and remuneration. A key factor in this regard for some individuals is a rejection of the appellation 'service user' as a derogatory and demeaning term. Peter Beresford (2005a) recognised the contentious nature of this and other terminology, but argued that, despite such problems, the term 'service user' may come to be a unifying concept for those concerned with rejecting negative connotations of identity and status, as part of a progressive movement.

As mentioned in Chapter 1, this territory is contested and politicised in a context of individuals and collective interest groups seeking to effect change. Politics for many service users is all about the art of the possible, about promoting change. A common feature of service users and carers who wish to become involved in universities, and for groups they may be affiliated to, is an expressed desire to in some way make a difference. Typically, people wish to contribute to changes in the provision of care services and encounters with professionals, beyond the confines of the campus or classroom. The university setting is seen as an important if indirect stepping stone for achieving these ends. Many also hold to broader personal and collective commitments to challenge prejudice, discrimination and disadvantage for a range of groups in society, often defined in terms of health or disability. The challenges are particularly concerned with how the wider political issues intersect with health and welfare institutions. Because of this, theory developed in the study of social movements and theorising emerging from within movements are useful means for reflecting on working practices, strategies of involvement and contention, and outcomes assessment, both positive and negative.

In everyday life, people do not typically think or express themselves in terms of formal theory. Nevertheless, a number of theoretical perspectives have been applied to understanding behaviour, motivation and reflections on self-hood and identity, including those concerned with distinctly personal or spiritual journeys. Much of the writing on social movements is concerned with the importance of human agency and creativity, and how this is worked out through the contribution of collective participation to a sense of community. Importantly, Barker and Cox (2002) distinguish between the external, academic study of movements and the knowledge about movements that is articulated by movement activists for themselves, with reference to Gramsci's (1971) distinction between *traditional* and *organic* intellectuals. These authors, both academics and activists themselves, recognise that a number of academics in the field of movement studies are drawn to it because of personal background in activism. There can be, however, tensions between academic interest in movements as objects of study and the more important issues for movement activists themselves concerning the theory and politics of action: what to do, and how best to do it (Cox and Fominaya, 2009). Theory is important for a number of reasons, not least its utility in supporting movements' attempts to frame and present their message, refute oppositional accounts, or critique the extent to which the status quo can be assumed to be immutable or grounded in common sense (Barker and Cox, 2002).

Theory developed for making sense of social movements, then, is arguably relevant to an interest in user and carer involvement. Many themes in this literature resonate with accounts which emerge from participants engaged in a range of involvement activity and community activism. The wider study of social movements aids understanding of questions exploring the nature of people's involvement. What motivates involvement in the first place? How do people become organised and what form does their organization take? What factors keep them going and sustain their involvement? How can participants' experiences be best understood? For movement activists, the answers to these questions have to move beyond dry academic concerns for explanation into thinking about how best to effect change.

2.2   New Social Movements

Ideas and activism focused on social change have latterly emerged in numerous collectives that have been described as new social movements, in contrast to more established groupings (Tarrow, 1998; Della Porta and Diani, 2006). Any collective means of pursuing social change can be thought of as a movement. Traditional social movements have included political parties and trade unions but, in the last few decades, the idea of 'new' social movements has taken hold (Beuchler, 2000). This concept suggests some key differences between the new and the old. In this critique, the older mass membership groups are taken to task for stifling the energy of activists within hierarchical and increasingly less democratic and co-opted forms of organization. For example, in the west the labour movement has latterly been criticised for a tendency towards bureaucratization, incorporation into the establishment, and relative political timidity (Hyman, 2007).

The newer movements are usually depicted as possessing greater vitality and radicalism, able to be expressed within flatter systems of democracy and sustained on the basis of relationships and friendships as much as the ability to forge a valued identity around a common purpose (Touraine, 1978; Melucci, 1996a; Klandermans, 1997). Furthermore, new social movements are said to be characterised by informal organization, membership from a wide social base, and engagement in new patterns of direct action (Wieviorka, 2005). Early examples in the United Kingdom include the Greenham Common peace protesters, the Twyford Down Dongas Camp and other anti-roads protests of the early and mid 1990s, and similar resistance to the expansion of airport runways. Other additions to the roll call of new social movements include Reclaim the Streets, protesters against genetic modification, and anti-capitalist and alter-globalization movements (Burgmann, 2003; Bramble and Minns, 2005; Carty and Onyett, 2006). The fact that these protest movements have minimal formal structure means they can come together when necessary, and then melt away (Klein, 2002). Frequently, such movements shun press coverage, preferring to publicise their objectives and activities via the Internet.

The alleged distinction between new and old social movements and associated debates are articulated at greater length elsewhere (Habermas, 1976, 1981; Crossley, 2002; Crossley and Roberts, 2004; Edwards, 2004, 2007, 2008). For the purpose of this chapter, it suffices to say at this juncture that organised service user movements have been recognised as part of this purported historical and conceptual shift (Rogers and Pilgrim, 1991; Brown and Zavetoski, 2005; Williamson, 2008). More recently, there has been concern that the distinction between old/bad and new/good is an artificial over-simplification, and that linkages and alliances between movements, however defined, are what matters most (Cresswell and Spandler, 2009; McKeown, 2009; Chapter 3, this volume).

Health and welfare user movements present resistance to the sort of institutionalised power represented by professional interests and authority. They also challenge the consequences of interaction between medical and social policy, wider governance, and personal and collective identity. Health inequalities, provision of services, access issues, and the contested territory of disease and disability, stigma, prejudice and discrimination are all opened up as targets for activism. This occurs within a more general disquiet with the increasingly privileged positioning of science and technology in society, and a critique of the linkage of broad socio-economic and political concerns with health (Brown and Zavetoski, 2005).

Service users and carers can be seen to have voice within a number of health and welfare movements, though the idea of a distinct carers movement has received much less attention than commentary on service users as a movement. For instance, in the history of psychiatric and mental health services there has always been a tradition of defending rights and entitlements and resisting or speaking out against oppressive practices (Campbell, 1996, 2009). A process of radicalization occurred in the 1970s (Spandler, 2006), and by the 1990s commentators were referring to organised service users as a new social movement (Rogers and Pilgrim, 1991; Crossley, 1999a, 1999b, 2006). More recently, those who use services, have survived services, or who choose not to use them, have arguably become more organised. A global disabled rights movement has existed since at least the 1980s (Oliver, 1990; Barton, 2001; Swain, French and Cameron, 2003) and has claimed to be the last civil rights movement (Driedger, 1989). The Direct Action Network is a group of disabled activists whose campaigns range over anti-institutionalization to improving access to public transport. The idea of a mental health service user movement alongside other such movements is now so well established that Crossley (2002) has recently questioned its 'newness'. The extent to which the idea of involvement and alliances have become an accepted part of mainstream policy and practice also raises the very real challenges of co-option and incorporation that have befallen previous movements, with the potential to dilute radical goals (Pilgrim, 2005; Campbell, 2009).

2.3 Movement Organization

The study of social movements has led to the articulation of various theoretical accounts which attempt to make sense of different organizational structures and the motivations of participants. These theories have emerged as part of wider critiques of late capitalism and globalization and the threats these pose for communities, citizen participation and control of the political economy. For Touraine (1978) a sense of identity in the movement emerges from individual capacity for self-reflective action, clarity of purpose and the focus of opposition. He contends that, for every historical period, social change is brought about by a particular movement, though it is not always apparent which movement this will be. Transformation occurs in a process whereby ideas for alternatives are created through action by individuals focused on specific aspects of society. This sense of 'what could be' mirrors the work of Habermas (1973). Patterns of industrialization, urbanization and development of communication technologies have led to profound changes and challenges for communities. Access to knowledge and information becomes a goal for movement activists and consumers alike (Castells, 1996, 1997, 1998), not least service users and carers.

Melucci connects identity formation with the production of meaning and self-realization in a context of participation in collective action. A stricter demarcation between private and public domains, seen in older movements, is dissolved in a more shifting, multi-faceted experience (Melucci, 1996b) where activism emerges from 'everyday life' (Melucci, 1996a: 114–115). Regardless of whether they start with a focus on identity, movements often create their own collective identity, often by way of rejecting those identities that would be imposed by others. For Castells, the very existence of the movement produces meaning for the activists and the wider community, regardless of any actual achievements.

Rothschild-Whitt (1979) described a number of identifying characteristics that differentiate new and old social movements. These include: rejection of hierarchical structures; decision making by consensus; absence of rules or central authority; sense of community; recruitment based upon relationships, friendships and shared values; egalitarian organization and sharing of tasks and roles. The primary incentive to become involved is usually common purpose. Solidarity and comradeship provide a secondary stimulus to join in. Material benefits feature some way down the list.

In a review of different theories, Klandermans (1997) suggested there are four main approaches to understanding movement organization, which he named:

- Symptom of institutionalization
- Resource mobilization
- Intrinsic goals
- Sponsors of meaning.

These are not meant to be taken as mutually exclusive or necessarily competing; rather, the various elements may figure differentially within or across movements at any time.

2.3.1   Symptom of Institutionalization

The existence of social grievances provides conditions for breakdown and the subsequent emergence of new social movements. Alienated individuals identify with and embrace the new organizations, but any replication of the sources of discontent, such as bureaucracy, formality and institutionalization, will undermine the movement and ultimately destroy it.

2.3.2 Resource Mobilization

Social movements are able to get going because necessary resources become available to communities. An important resource is the actual system of organization and being organised is a means of securing power or achieving goals. The operation of social movements involves garnering and distributing resources, including those supplied by individuals or institutional supporters. Individuals, in this analysis, make rational decisions whether to support or join the movement based on personal costs or benefits of doing so.

2.3.3 Intrinsic Goals

The organization becomes a goal in itself. In an alternative to a strategic viewpoint, this concerns the process by which a sense of common identity and solidarity are brought into being in movements (Cohen, 1985). This perspective is critical of some features of rational choice implicit in resource mobilization theories. These theories are criticised for taking for granted the existence of the social movement organization, which is the very thing that others seek to explain.

2.3.4 Sponsors of Meaning

This perspective draws on symbolic interactionist sociology, constructionist theories and cultural aspects of new social movements to focus on the role of such organizations as sponsors of meaning. The notion of 'framing' has become prominent in this body of work, starting with Goffman (1974) and developed by various movement scholars to reflect the means by which movement activists interpret the world, make sense of their circumstances and precipitate thinking about alternative possibilities and solutions (Donati, 1992; Snow and Benford, 1988). Gusfield (1970), one of the earlier commentators on the development of collective meanings, remarked: *'What comes to be seen as injustice must be pointed to, named and described from amongst the logically possible interpretations for the potential adherents' sense of discontent'*.

2.4 Individuality, Community and Prefigurative Politics

Consideration of the various forms of voluntarism and community and movement activism can illustrate interesting dimensions of personal motivation, especially at the juncture of individuality and collectivism. Theories drawn from different traditions can assist developing a richer understanding of these matters. Over a number of years, the American social psychologist Batson and his colleagues (Batson, Ahmad and Tsang, 2002) have explored the nature of people's motivation to get involved in community activities. They describe four categories of motivation: egoistic, to benefit one-self; altruistic, to benefit another individual; collectivistic, to benefit a group; and principled, grounded in values or to uphold a moral principle. These authors acknowledge that it is an accepted orthodoxy in western society that human behaviour is goal directed and primarily motivated by self-interest. Though this selfish impulse certainly does exist, they reject the idea that it is all encompassing and propose that any adequate analysis of actions for the common good must include the other sources of motivation. The suggested categories of motivation can subsume complexities of feelings. Altruism, for example, may involve empathic responses to individuals, or be inspired by guilt at the thought of doing nothing.

From a sociological perspective, Delanty (2003) contrasts the sort of individualism that might support collectivism and activism in social movements with the singularly self-interested individual of new-right political thinking. In Delanty's analysis, such individualism combines personal self-fulfilment with commitment to action and achievement of shared goals. The activists have their personalism or selfhood shaped in a construction of community that arises in the act of mobilizing the movement towards transformative goals; individual agency, energy and creativity are important, contributing to but ultimately transcended in collective participation. These ideas connect with the more progressive thinking on social capital, especially as applied to the distribution of community and movement resources (Jarley, 2005; Chapter 3, this volume).

The creative individuality that Delanty (2003) recognises in community collectivism is similarly evident in consideration of service user and carer contributions to teaching or research. The way in which people draw on their own experiences of ill health and use of services to render this meaningful in students' learning is a significant creative act. William Park (Chapter 10) takes this point further and argues that lay teachers can transcend a personal history of health difficulties in the act of asserting their own unique capacity for creativity, resilience and self-belief. In doing so, the resultant communicative act can be a vehicle for challenging stigma relating to ill health or disability and, in relation to mental health, align itself with progressive notions of recovery (Pilgrim, 2008).

A relevant theme in the discourse of social movement activists and scholars alike is the notion of prefigurative politics. Prefiguration describes the way people in social movements try to practise what they preach in trialling their ideals for alternative futures in the actual mechanisms of transition. They have a vision for a future world and, in the act of trying to realise it, they try to model what it is they are trying to achieve. Put more simply, this is about the *means* of achieving a new social order being as important as the *ends*. These ideas can be attributed to various sources, from the theological to humanistic strands of Marxism or various anarchist philosophies. Prefigurative themes can be ascertained in the writings of the Italian Marxist Antonio Gramsci (Gramsci, 1971; Golding, 1992), but Burton and Kagan (2007) also see resonance with Paolo Freire's (1999) humanist notion of untested feasibility. Anarchist scholars and activists working within contemporary social movements have done much to develop the idea of prefigurative politics (Day, 2005), and connect with a long tradition of utopian thinking and communities grounded in affinity for fellows and consensus decision taking.

William Park (Chapter 10) connects prefigurative ideas with the humanism evident in the writings of Abraham Maslow (1994) and Paolo Freire (1971). Each
in their own way, these authors offer insights into emancipatory journeys for
participants in education. Maslow emphasises the objective of individual self-
actualization, whilst Freire stresses collective liberation, but both see facilitative,
experiential learning as crucial. It is not surprising then that Freire's ideas have
been inspirational within social movements and associated with the development
of progressive models of action learning and participatory or emancipatory action
research.

Prefigurative politics are arguably most often evident in the means for taking
collective decisions and the positive quality of relationships between activists. In
their reflections on the transformative potential in various settings, Burton and
Kagan (2007) highlight the struggle between prefigurative models for social
change and forces for reaction and conservatism. Drawing on late 1960s radicalism and feminism, Kris Rondeau of the Harvard Union of Clerical and Technical
Workers, for instance, developed a relational approach to trade union activism,
organizing mainly low paid women workers in this prestigious United States
University (Hoerr, 1997). This proved to be a profoundly successful style of union
organization that emphasised kindness in relationships with both colleagues and
adversaries. The quality of relationships is the primary focus, over and above
attention to workplace issues. Once established, the attendant solidarity enables
an empowered response to particular issues, and lowers dependence upon
union officials. Interestingly, once an effective university union was established,
Rondeau and colleagues turned their attention to organizing in the local hospital
and commenced building alliances with self-organised service user groups, under
the slogan 'pro-patient, pro-union'.

2.5   Involvement as a Movement?

There are some clear resonances between research and commentary on health
and social care service user involvement and the wider literature on social movements (Chapter 9). If the involvement of service users and carers within universities does have transformative features or potential, then emerging organizational
forms may very well prefigure progressive turns in the politics of health, disability
and academia itself. This connects with the work of Pelias (2004: 1–2) who argues
for new ways of working in academia:

> I never want to hurt or be hurt, but too often I have watched claims of truth try to tri-
> umph over compassion, try to crush alternative possibilities and try to silence minority
> voices. Seeing the pain this causes, I seek another discourse, one that still has an edge,
> that could say what needs to be said but would do no harm. I want a scholarship that
> fosters connections, opens spaces for dialogue, heals. I want to rein in power like one
> might a runaway horse. I need to write from the heart.

The rise of health-focused social movements can be explained by a number of factors, including a resistance to the hegemony of medical power and its influence on decision making and policy framing (Brown and Zavetoski, 2005). In the last decade, this has been wrapped up in the fashion for evidence-based medicine, but is also part of wider social trends that conjoin appeals to scientific understanding with social governance and regulation. Health social movements have sought better services and challenged the primacy of medical expertise, highlighting limitations of knowledge and resisting the creeping medicalization of a range of social problems. This often translates into resistance to medical authority, identified by some as another wing of the exercise of state power. Social movements offer both a critique of existing structures, and alternative ways of constructing reality.

Involvement initiatives within universities are one space where the user movement might make inroads; with the important caveat that incorporation threats are clearly present.

Such involvement initiatives present opportunities for bringing about social change and need not be hindered by a direct association with service provision. An emphasis on solidarity and common purpose is clearly related to making a difference in practice. Participation in such endeavours can be seen to be both an end and a means to an end. Touraine's declaration that for each historical period there is one social movement that brings about transformative change might be accomplished in our time by the wider user and carers' movement. Better yet if this can be achieved in progressive alliances with staff (McKeown and Spandler, 2006).

Service user and carer participants in university settings ought not only be defined in terms of particular health or disability experiences. They bring forward their complete personalities, their talents and creative strengths, personal worldviews, philosophies and spiritual beliefs. Resonant with Delanty's (2003) community spirited individualism, an unselfish respect for common humanity and concern for others is key, but alongside this the conditions for self-actualization for participants are perceptible. Freire's (1971) model for participatory learning and development provides a common philosophy to underpin both the development of models of user and carer involvement and approaches to teaching and learning for university students.

Service users, carers and university personnel working collaboratively can assume different identities. True partnership can offer up positive identities of self-respect in a context of critical awareness and altruistic regard for others. As this partnership advances, traditional hierarchies of status and esteem are open for transformation, and this may threaten valued aspects of academic identity for some staff. The actualization of alternative ways of being, however, presents the potential for more positive and wholesome identities all round. For service users and carers, superimposed and negative identity can be discarded. University personnel can assume the identity of critically engaged academics, with their positive contribution to communities recognised and valued (Spandler and McKeown, 2008; Chapter 3, this volume).

The accounts drawn on here demonstrate that radical visions for alternative futures and the popular protest needed to achieve them continue to survive into contemporary times in a range of social movements and community activism, with health and welfare user movements being a particularly interesting example. This chapter has reflected on the extent to which these movements can become insinuated into the practices of universities, and how involvement in these developments can affect the experiences of participants. This is not to go so far as to suggest that service user and carer involvement within university settings is a fully-fledged radical movement, or that participants are all conscious activists for change. For example, involvement in universities may have more in common with patterns of community voluntarism rather it does with politicised movements. Furthermore, 'involvement' initiatives that bring self-organised groups and independent individuals into public institutions almost inevitably suffer a process of co-option and dilution of independence and radical objectives. There is a need to think clearly about the differences between a *user movement* and *user involvement*, without overly romanticizing the latter as an example of the former. Barker and Cox's (2002: 22) observation is relevant here:

> Movement activists are not the Robinson Crusoes presented by individualist rationalisms, nor the beings of pure thought presented by idealist constructivisms. It might be more appropriate to think of them as people who do not always *know* what needs are driving them, but who are engaged in *finding out*, through struggle and through solidarity. (*emphasis* in the original)

There are commonalities and cross-overs between involvement initiatives and social movements, and insights from movement knowledge developed in other contexts can assist participants in this process of *finding out*, making decisions and strategies. This is especially germane in those circumstances where tensions are exposed between the institutional interests of universities and the more radical claims of participants, including those associated with important differentials in power, status and remuneration. Parr (2008: 28) has highlighted the contribution an understanding of social space can make to exploring the transition mental health service users can make from a devalued identity framed around illness to the more 'valued and relational social agent'. It may be the case that the ultimate success of involvement initiatives in university settings herald profound implications for human relationships within health and social care services and, indeed, issues of common identity and humanity for us all (further exploration of this point is given in Chapter 5). This has the potential, in the long run, to lead to the dismantling of constructions of social difference framed around illness and disability, and the forms of systemic disadvantage which flow from this.

These themes are taken up further in Chapter 9, which makes connections between the experiences and narratives of service users and carers engaged in the Comensus initiative and the theoretical accounts of movements, motivations and mobilization presented here.

3 Beyond the Campus: Universities, Community Engagement and Social Enterprise

I started with the university four years ago and felt dwarfed by my lack of intellect, but over the years I have been met with warmth by academics and made new friends with lots of wonderful caring people who have broadened my horizons. My life is full and happy.

3.1 Introduction

Service user and carer involvement in universities sits within, and is supported by, a whole raft of wider community engagement, some connected to the university, some not. This endeavour comprises self-organised groups in a panoply of civic spirit, voluntarism and so-called 'third-sector' activity that has a life of its own beyond the campus. As seen in Chapter 2, the idea of user and carer groups as a social movement fits within this configuration. Universities themselves can potentially play a key role in supporting these community efforts for the common good, establishing themselves as civically engaged institutions.

Commentators from a variety of theoretical perspectives have pondered the need to develop ways of thinking about these social and pro-social forms differently from orthodox theorizing developed to fit the world of business and markets. Theories of social capital have been put forward to account for the processes, effects and value at stake in these rich relationships and networks. The fact that community-orientated work might be organised in ways that harness characteristics of enterprise and entrepreneurship has latterly come together in hybrid social enterprises and social firms. These organizations are a small but growing contributor to national economies, and provide one set of opportunities to harness the creativity of activists, cascade benefits into communities and promote employability amongst service user groups typically excluded from mainstream labour markets. Similarly, models of social marketing are now operated, including significant contributions to health promotion.

In this chapter we first look at the range of civic engagement that can exist in communities regardless of university involvement. We then turn to address the many ways in which universities have become more reciprocally engaged with their local communities and explore the possibilities that open up, including challenges to academic identity and the realization of new roles for critically engaged academics in alliance with community groups. Social enterprises and social firms are then reflected upon as a potential route to establishing independence for service users and carers actively engaged with universities, possibly minimizing co-option and incorporation threats. Social marketing will be considered as an interesting development which brings together many of these themes. In our conclusions we home in on the experience of alienation in professional encounters with service users as a point of departure to promote alliance as an important source of better experiences for users and carers, and improved fulfilment in job role for health and social care practitioners and academics alike.

3.2 Communities

Before thinking about ideas of community and civic engagement, it is worth considering that for some the very idea of community is a contested concept. For others, even when the notion of community is more or less accepted, the term can mean different things to different people. A community can be thought of in a number of ways, being defined variously as a geographically located area or place, or as a collection of people held together by common interest, ethnicity, culture or faith, for example. In arriving at agreed definitions of community, the interplay between sense of place and socio-cultural factors can be complex.

Margaret Thatcher once famously derided the idea of 'society' to make the point that, in her view, in the arena of politics and economics the self-interested individual, largely separated from neighbours or fellows, reigned supreme. It has been seen, in Chapter 2, how this perspective has been challenged by a generation of scholars concerned with the effects of globalization and urbanization, asserting the continued value of thinking about the interconnectedness of people in communities and how these can bring into being the different ways in which people see themselves and are seen by others. Here the work of Delanty (2003) is particularly interesting, as he suggests that some of the attributes that are most usually thought of as belonging to the individualism of new right political science are just as much characteristic of the fellowships and associations of communal life. These are very much brought to life through participation in community and civic engagement.

Delanty (2003) describes how early theories of communitarianism located individualism as the enemy of community – undermining civic pride, social capital and voluntarism. He proposes, however, that we can conceive of a new individualism that supports and sustains community and collective action:

> Personal self-fulfilment and individualised expression can be highly compatible with collective participation . . . Community can be a means of releasing the cultural reactivity that late modernity produces but does not fully exploit . . . people from diverse backgrounds can come together in communal activism united by a common commitment and the solidarity that results. (Delanty, 2003: 120, 122)

Meegan and Mitchell (2001), focusing on 'neighbourhood renewal' as a form of urban regeneration and social inclusion policy, consider the different ways in which notions of community can be conceived by policy makers and community members. Drawing on previous reviews by Davies and Herbert (1993) they describe seven selected definitions which incorporate notions of geographical place and socio-cultural features (Box 3.1).

Box 3.1   Different Notions of Community or Neighbourhood

- Simple neighbourly contact and proximity as the basis for informal organization grounded in local interests and sentiment.
- A distinct territorial group reflecting the physical characteristics of the area and social characteristics of the inhabitants.
- Areas which are distinctive in terms of four elements: clear boundaries; ethnic or cultural characteristics of residents; a sense of people belonging together; local use of facilities for shopping, leisure and so on. However, areas containing all four elements might be hard to find.
- Areas with a strong sense of shared history and local awareness of interests; may include a set of local organizations and businesses.
- The collective life and institutional arrangements of a community is its definition, implying shared interests and norms of behaviour.
- Self-definition: the community or neighbourhood is what people say it is.
- Community as the sum of social relationships and interconnections by which people express shared interest in the local society. Not a place, but place focused activity.

Adapted from Meegan and Mitchell (2001: 2173). Reproduced by permission of Sage Publications

---

3.3 Community Engagement

A variety of terms (community engagement, civic engagement, community organizing, movement organizing) have been applied to the sort of participatory grass roots activity of groups and organizations seeking some sense of common good. This sort of thing can be seen in one form or another almost anywhere one cares to look for it. Barack Obama's own personal involvement in community activism for the Gamaliel Foundation in Chicago has received significant attention in the global media, highlighting the positive contribution to civic society made by such individuals and groups. Furthermore, Obama's election team freely adopted lessons learnt from experience in community organizing to assist in mobilizing the vote in the US presidential election.

Various authors have been interested in the extent to which community engagement is informally political in character, concerned with social change, or leads to involvement in formal political process such as electoral politics, local and national government (Ball, 2005; Hays, 2007). The social movements' literature suggests that any engagement with political and legal infrastructure can be either consensual or driven by conflict. The state and various public institutions might (possibly for different reasons) also be interested in community or public engagement, and these grass roots groups can find themselves sought after to engage with government, service industries and organizations such as universities. The contemporary popularity of theories of social capital (Section 3.4) has led many governments to focus at a community level for solutions to social inequalities and disadvantage, often under the conceptual umbrella of social inclusion. For anarchists, such as Day (2005), the purely social form of activism eschews involvement in political or state structures, and the relationships and fellowships forged in activism are the engine for change, prefiguring a new politics of affinity.

Civic engagement takes numerous forms and covers a wide range of issues, including (but not exhaustively) those with a focal point on:

- Environmental concerns
- Urban regeneration
- Rights and legal issues
- Trade unions and social movements
- Community arts and culture
- Health and public health initiatives
- Disaster relief and response to catastrophes
- International development, including international health initiatives around disease prevention, for example HIV/AIDS.

Various universities and individual scholars can be seen to have supported or become involved in all of these forms (Section 3.8) as part of their own university's community engagement programmes, or led by personal interest.

Participation in community level activities can lead to numerous positive effects within communities and for individuals, beyond the realization of particular goals and objectives for specific groups. Some of these positive effects can occur without the group actually achieving its original aims. For example, grass roots efforts can help to build healthier communities and the capability for people to begin to state for themselves what is important to them and their community (Fawcett, Fransisco and Paine-Andrews, 2000). In the immediate aftermath of the 9/11 atrocity in New York, Steffen and Fothergill (2009) observed a massive, spontaneous community response. On reflection, they were able to describe the positive effects for volunteers in regard to their own journeys of recovery from the trauma of this attack on their community.

The fact that there is a wealth of participatory activity within communities does not hide the fact that not everyone either wishes, or is able, to participate. Price (2002) contends that people wishing to be engaged and help their communities can be blocked by a range of structural barriers that limit opportunities. Once people are involved as community activists they can face a struggle to resist co-option into formal or institutional structures (Whelan and Lyons, 2005). Bond and colleagues (2008) point out that women are under-represented in formal civic roles but permeate informal grass roots systems of organizing and community groups, neighbourhood and community movements. They manage this despite various other demands on their time. In a case study of the attitudes of civically active people in one US city, Hays (2007) found that community activists are both critical of those people who do not participate and frustrated at not being able to involve more people.

Hays (2007) also observed that people who engaged in community volunteering or joined community-based groups and associations were often also involved in political engagement, aimed at influencing policy or electoral outcomes. Though these two forms of activism were linked, the participants saw them differently and obtained different rewards from each. Many saw the formal political context as an arena of conflict, whereas their community involvement was typically co-operative. Hays (2007) goes on to bemoan the institutional constraints upon true democratic participation in the United States, notably the concentration of power and economic advantage in elites, which people are often unaware of. Another barrier to more complete involvement is that the political elites are nervous of increased participation because of uncertainty or unpredictability about where it will all lead. Hays (2007: 423) argues for the creation of 'public spaces' for 'meaningful political connections . . . and action on the part of ordinary citizens', which wouldn't overturn the prevailing constraints but would represent a very different model of democracy.

In Chapter 2 the literature on social movements was reviewed; much of it can be thought of as being part of a broad politics of contention, where, at the very least, community involvement is about the marginalised and disadvantaged making demands on the powerful. Sirianni and Friedland (2001) have analysed some of the complexities of power conflict and opposition at stake in community empowerment. They argue that at least some of the language of groups concerned with civic renewal in the United States is very much about consensus formation and finding common ground. Though this is not as simple as saying this activism is singularly forged around consensus, neither does it fit neatly an uncomplicated framing of oppositional politics. Some of the relational and prefigurative elements of internal movement discourse, such as the development of horizontal democracy, also involve consensus decision making, without forgetting that participants are clearly operating from a standpoint of opposition. From the completely different perspective of institutional development of systems of public participation or consultation, the uncertainty and unpredictability of unfettered engagement can be minimised by efforts to promote consensus (Ashcraft, 2007). Ashcraft describes a number of strategies for the 'management' of public meetings, including independent facilitation, convergence strategies and dot polling. Despite the unsettling managerial tone, many of these and similar strategies are already adopted by independent community groups for building their own consensus.

3.4   The Contested Concept of Social Capital

Undoubtedly, the rich networks of mutuality, reciprocity, cooperation and support that are evident in forms of voluntarism, civic and community activism and social movements are almost by definition pro-social in effect and deeply social in character. This characteristic of community sustains itself in a myriad of ways, but common features include dynamic individuals with a commitment to a sense of common good interacting with each other in mutually rewarding relationships and friendships which extend into multifarious networks and connection within and between groups. The idea that there is some personal and collective value in this sort of community connectedness or networking has been referred to as 'social capital'. The author who has done most to popularise the term is Robert Putnam (2000). In his *Bowling Alone: The Collapse and Revival of American Community*, Putnam argues that aspects of social capital have declined in US communities, and this demise of civic engagement helps to explain social disorder. Putnam acknowledges that the term has been around for some time, but cites Jane Jacobs (1961) and James Coleman (1988) as originators of the current usage of the concept and key developer of theory, respectively. Relevant and influential themes and theorizing are also to be found in the earlier work of Alexis de Tocqueville (1966) and Pierre Bourdieu (1977, 1986).

Putnam (2000) and others have been criticised for neglecting to consider power, class and inequality, issues of victim blaming and the potential exclusionary tactics of some tightly connected communities in their theorizing on social capital. Various authors (Jarley, 2005; Hyman, 2007), while critical of Putnam's treatment of the idea, have been interested in presenting a more progressive or transformational conceptualisation of social capital.

Jarley (2005), for instance, in a context of UK trade union renewal, is highly critical of patterns of 'servicing', whereby rank and file members become increasingly dependent on full-time officers. These developments prompt objections in view of their apparent deviation from the sorts of mutual support associated with traditional models of trade union organizing. One solution is to build up the role played by lay activists, but this can risk overburdening them. A remedy lies in expanding and strengthening social capital within the union, involving both internal and external relationships (Jarley, 2005; Saundry, Stuart and Antcliff, 2008). Such an approach would bring together mutual support across a range of issues, including non-workplace or community objectives. This form of collectivism heralds opportunities for a creative nexus between community interests and trade union activity (Cranford and Ladd, 2003; Wills and Simms, 2004; McKeown, 2009). With reference to earlier work by Law and Mooney (2006), Richard Hyman (2007: 12) further develops these ideas to suggest that a form of 'insurgent social capital' could be brought forward in 'broad networks of mutuality' so that unions are in a better position to resist the 'remorseless drive of neo-liberalism'. In a similar vein, Healy and Meagher (2004) bemoan the undermining of public value for human services work, particularly in the case of social work, and offer a collective solution that makes the most of new models of professionalism and trade unionism.

These ideas have led to the development of an organizing model called 'reciprocal community unionism'. Trade unions support community campaigns and the community supports union campaigns. Examples of alliances of this sort have come together over single issues such as the Living Wage Campaign. Hyman (2007) argues that trade unions can reclaim themselves as campaigning organizations concerned with politics of contention. They can also put aside internecine tensions that divide them, find outlets for cooperative activism around common causes and attempt to build new democratic relationships between activists and leadership, and workers and service users. We all have a stake in forging broadly based community alliances in advance of any dispute or campaign, so that solidarity can be assumed rather than built from scratch every time it is needed (Wills and Simms, 2004).

The Health sector of Unison[1] is currently piloting a 'relational' model of organizing in one branch in the South Eastern region of England, based upon the experiences of the Harvard Union of Clerical and Technical Workers and inspired by feminist ideas (Hoerr, 1997). This builds solidarity and empowers members based on a foundation of workplace connections, friendships and resourcefulness. Other Unison activities, notably around the Living Wage Campaign and London Citizens, suggest a growing affinity for connecting with coalitions of community activism (Unison, 2008; Littman, 2008; Wills, 2007; Bayley, 2006).

3.5   Social Enterprise and Social Entrepreneurship

Akin to the way in which the concept of social capital has been articulated to differentiate its social character from other forms, such as material or cultural capital, recent times have witnessed significant practical and scholarly interest in the term 'social enterprise', adopted to signify economic activity with social objectives (Mayo, 2002; Leadbeater, 2002; Pearce, 2003; Morrin, Simmonds and Somerville, 2004; Nyssens, 2006; Chell, 2007; Mason, Kirkbride and Bryde, 2007; Zografos, 2007). Similarly, the language of 'social entrepreneurship' and 'social marketing' has been coined to recognise that this sort of business-like activity can also be organised to address social benefit for communities. There seems to be no end

---

[1] A UK public service trade union.

to the capacity for neologizing with Dixon and Clifford's (2007) notion of 'eco-preneurship' to define entrepreneurs acting in defence of ecological concerns.

The United Kingdom government (DTI, 2002: 7) describes a social enterprise as:

> a business with primarily social objectives whose surpluses are principally re-invested for that purpose in the business or in the community, rather than being driven by the need to realise profit for shareholders.

Actual social enterprises can take many forms, depending on how broadly or narrowly they are defined. Morrin and colleagues (2004) note 20 distinct forms on an expansive definition of the term. They also note that the recent positive recognition afforded social enterprise is reflected in increasing levels of government support and interest and systems of grant allocation and awards ceremonies for notable success stories. The rise in favour of social enterprise was marked with a special supplement of New Statesman magazine, celebrating the phenomenon (Mayo, 2002; Leadbeater, 2002).

Notwithstanding its recent popularity, it is possible that the admixture of business and social orientations is not a completely new phenomenon. Shaw (2004), in an overview and discussion of social entrepreneurship, traces the history back to the nineteenth century and the likes of Robert Owen with his model workplace and community at New Lanark Mill in Scotland. Similarly, the cooperative form has a lengthy and sometimes illustrious history (Birchall, 1997). Morrin and colleagues (2004) wryly observe that earlier examples of social enterprise remained largely hidden, even in the 1980s and 1990s, because they stood outside of prevailing economic orthodoxy. Kerlin (2006) highlights differences in the concept across the globe and within regions. She notes that within Europe social enterprises have largely focused on those areas that the state has retreated from.

There is a growing literature that discusses features of this business model, including valuable commentary on systems for governance and legal frameworks (Mason, Kirkbride and Bryde, 2007; Ridley-Duff, 2007). Morrin and colleagues (2004) offer a number of case studies of successful United Kingdom examples of social enterprises from which others can hope to learn. Other publications offer more detailed guidance on the practicalities of how to initiate a social enterprise (Pearce, 2003). The majority of publications are broadly in favour of social enterprise, though there are some counterblasts (Dart, 2004; Schofield, 2005). For Leadbeater (2002), it is the tension between social goals and commercial imperatives that makes these organizations potentially highly innovative.

A number of authors have remarked upon the difficulties social enterprises face in securing either start-up finance or in achieving sustainability beyond public funding or grant capture (Harding, 2007). Arguably, they do not differ in this regard from other not-for-profit and voluntary sector organizations. For Chell (2007), the typical survival strategy for social enterprises lies in securing grant funding or government money. To become more entrepreneurial and self-sustaining requires a re-conceptualisation of the notion of entrepreneurship to include creation of social benefit or value together with economic value. In a context of corporate responsibility, this new view of entrepreneurship could also apply to private firms.

At a more practical level, it has been persuasively suggested that new sources of finance need to be organised to better support social enterprises.

Buttle (2008) argues for new types of social finance organizations to lend to social enterprises, highlighting the case of the Charity Bank. Similarly, Lewis (2009) welcomes the UK government Office of the Third Sector proposals for a new social investment bank, but asserts that any new organization would have to be significantly different from a typical bank. At least one of its tasks would be to raise the profile and attractiveness of investment in social enterprises, so that they become a consideration of any potential financier looking for somewhere to invest their money. In a similar vein, Pepin (2005) offers an account of philanthropic donations in the United States plugging the gap in finances for social enterprises and other third sector groups.

The internal organization of social enterprises, particularly systems of governance, has been a focus of interest (Mason, Kirkbride and Bryde, 2007; Ridley-Duff, 2007) with some analyses linked to notions of legitimacy (Dart, 2004). For Mason and colleagues (2007), governance arrangements need to take account of social enterprise as a social institution, where wider groups of stakeholders affected by the activity of the organization have a claim on resources, without having a direct financial stake in it. The fact that communities contain people who can both affect the particular social enterprise organization or be affected by it ought to be in some way reflected in governance structures. More radical models for governance that take account of this multiplicity of community stakeholders are proposed by Ridley-Duff (2007) grounded in inclusive democratic principles (Section 3.6). Conversely, a constellation of external pressures, including regulatory requirements, but also the presentation of best practice examples to slavishly follow, is possibly leading to a form of institutional 'isomorphism' with a lack of differentiation in governance structures (Mason, Kirkbride and Bryde, 2007). Burrows (2004) noted the arrival of legislation in the United Kingdom for the introduction of Community Interest, and subsequent criticism from the voluntary sector that this move might diminish rather than enhance a pluralistic diversity of service providers; restricting social enterprises to a single, newly created sector.

For Rothschild (2009), the cooperative model extends a form of democracy into the economic/work sphere that could translate into greater confidence for participation into other realms, both civic and political. Less optimistically, Cornelius and colleagues (2008) note that some employees of social enterprises have experienced similar disgruntlement with terms and conditions, management and job dissatisfaction to those experienced working in a standard business. Connecting with ideas around corporate responsibility, these authors contend that the negative experiences of certain employees of social enterprises go against the values implicit in progressive social missions. They suggest that the internal affinity for employee welfare can become lost within outward looking practices focused on social concerns.

From a critical standpoint, other commentators take a negative view of the conflation of ideologies inherent in the notion of social enterprise, and have divined reluctance amongst participants or beneficiaries to fully embrace the language and concepts of the business world. Froggett and Chamberlayne (2004), for example, criticise the terminology of social enterprise and social entrepreneurship, questioning its adequacy for characterising people's community activism. Similarly, the managerially defined shift towards an enterprise culture is questioned by Parkinson and Howorth (2008), whose discourse analytic study found that the language used by those grass roots people identified as social entrepreneurs did not fit easily with the prevailing business rhetoric. They were more likely to construct themselves and their associated activity in terms of localism and social morality.

Dart (2004) expresses a worry that, over time, moral legitimacy will be lost because the business philosophy will swallow up the potential for innovatory prosocial organization and social enterprises might eventually evolve into firms that are narrowly market orientated, commercial and revenue seeking like any others. For him this potential is evident because of a connection between the recent focus on social enterprise and reactionary ideologies of neo-liberalism and privatization.

A general retreat from the State in western democracies has also begun to associate the growth of social enterprise with the operation of existing public services. In the United Kingdom, the policy white paper *Our health, Our care, Our Say* (DH, 2006a) identified social enterprise as a means of introducing diversity into public service provision. In the light of this, many practitioners and their trade unions have voiced concerns about fragmentation of existing community services, employee job security, deviation from the stated goals of user empowerment towards more iniquitous business goals and opening up the sector to more predatory full-blown privatizations (Cook, 2006; Marks and Hunter, 2007). Context is important, however, and O'Toole and Burdess (2004) describe how social enterprises in Australian outback communities took over local government agencies and institutions when the state pulled out from providing them. Questions arise over the extent to which these might now lack the sort of legitimacy and accountability associated with electoral process, but this is tempered by the acknowledgement that without these social enterprises many small towns would simply not have survived.

The Economist (2005) wryly notes that critical concerns surrounding the direction of policy on social enterprise will not be diminished by the fact in the United Kingdom that both main political parties are strong supporters: Labour as part of wider public sector 'reform', and Conservatives as a means to bypass local bureaucracies. Bell (2001) goes further in a paper titled *Imagining Marketopia*, asserting that application of market ideologies to all aspects of life would create a world where nothing has intrinsic value any more.

Morrin and colleagues (2004) suggest that, despite many excellent examples of social enterprise, the jury is out on whether there is any measurable impact on the economy as a whole. A bigger economic impact may result if there is a real shift to delivering public services, but the resultant organizations might prove to have 'borrowed the form of social enterprise, if not the heart' (Morrin *et al.*, 2004: 74).

3.6   Involving Service Users: the Social Firm

A development in the field of social enterprise has been the establishment of organizations whose social benefit purpose involves provision of employment for those marginalised and excluded from mainstream labour markets. This includes people in health and social care service user groups such as the disabled or those with enduring mental health problems. Indeed, an early example of use of the term social enterprise came from Italy where social businesses created employment opportunities for mental health service users (De Leonardis and Mauri, 1992). These initiatives were linked to Italian deinstitutionalization experiences, and were heavily influenced by Basaglia and the Italian anti-psychiatry movement (Ducci, Stentella and Vulterini, 2002). In the United Kingdom, social enterprises that take this form have come to be known as social firms and have been supported by the network *Social Firms UK* (www.socialfirms.co.uk). Across Europe, social enterprises concerned with increasing access to employment, bringing in the traditionally long-term unemployed as well as disability groups, have been afforded the acronym WISE – work integration social enterprises – and these have often been constituted as cooperatives (Nyssens, 2006). There is also a pan-European Confederation of Social Firms (Ducci, Stentella and Vulterini, 2002).

Ducci and colleagues (2002: 76–78) suggest the following criteria for classifying an enterprise as a social firm:

- A business created for employment of people with a disability or other disadvantage in the labour market.
- It uses market-orientated production of goods or services to pursue its social mission.
- A significant number of its employees will be people with a disability or other disadvantage in the labour market.
- All workers are paid the market rate wage or salary appropriate to the work, whatever their productive capacity.
- Work opportunities should be equal between disadvantaged and non-disadvantaged employees. All employees have the same employment rights and obligations.

Mancino and Thomas (2005), reviewing social enterprise in Italy, describe a successful but fragile model because of legislative uncertainties and over-reliance on public funding. They make the point that systems of grant allocation favour low cost tenders over aspiration for high quality service provision. In a wider European review, Ducci, Stentella and Vulterini (2002: 76) remark upon the 'motley array of legislation norms, organizational forms and conceptual models' necessitating any definition to be broadly drawn. They state that it is imperative to find jobs within social firms that suit the characteristics of their disadvantaged members and, at the same time, meet the demands of the market.

In an Italian study of 420 members of a single cooperative by Savio and Righetti (1993), the two largest groups were users of social services and mental health service users. A high turnover rate amongst the workforce was interpreted as indicating the role that cooperatives play as a stepping stone on route to more desirable and rewarding employment in the mainstream labour market. In line with the general literature on social enterprises, there is a question mark over sustainability beyond grant funding for social firms (Phillips, 2006) coupled with concerns that some initiatives lack independence from statutory services (Ducci, Stentella and Vulterini, 2002). Spear and Bidet's (2005) review of European initiatives found that work integration for marginalised groups is an effective form of social enterprise, but questions remain about how best to maintain activity and spread best practice.

Ridley-Duff (2007) argues that one answer to the sustainability question lies in attention to the governance structures for social firms. Democratic control of social enterprises based upon a communitarian model is proposed, such that they are owned and controlled by their beneficiaries or employees. The Community Interest Company (CIC) model and enabling legislation do not insist that directors pay attention to the views of different stakeholders who must have faith that these businesses will be run ethically for the common good. The communitarian philosophy is proposed as an alternative to the prevailing unitarian form, opening up the possibilities for pluralistic systems of governance, at once more democratic and participatory, and more likely because of this to lead to greater sustainability. 'The most enduring impacts are likely to come from organizations that tackle social exclusion on both fronts – embracing a trading purpose that addresses the perceived needs of socially excluded groups and allowing participation by them in decision making and wealth creating processes' (Ridely-Duff, 2007: 390).

3.7   Community, Service User and Practitioner Alliances

There is a tradition within health and social care services of critically engaged practitioners playing a role in community engagement and politics, and forging alliances with the user movement and other groups in defence of services (Spandler, 2006; McKeown, 2009; Cox 2009). This sort of activity is often associated with efforts to refashion professional identity and escape the trappings of outmoded archetypes of professionalism (Davies, 1995; Healy, 2000; Salvage, 2002). Haynes and White (1999) call for social work in the United States to stand for a range of progressive causes, including community engagement. Powell and Geoghegan (2005: 139) go further to argue that social workers should embrace internationalism and take on a global role. They deny that this amounts to a form of 'ethical welfare imperialism' and take up a view of community as 'we' rather than 'me, myself alone'. Their blueprint for practice includes user participation and empowerment as one of ten key principles, and they see alliances between community groups and the enabling state: 'it is in these interstices that social work can find a distinctive professional mission that promotes the values that it espouses and empowers those it has traditionally sought to serve' (Powell and Geoghegan, 2005:143). A manifesto for a critically engaged social work practice, written by practitioners and academics in the United Kingdom, helped to launch a radical social work movement, the Social Work Action Network, grounded in principles of social justice and engagement (Jones *et al.*, 2004).

Commentary on campaigning to establish the National Health Service, and struggles to defend it from cuts or closures, indicates that practitioner and service user political alliances have always potentiated a debate about who has a say in decision making and control of services (Doyal, 1979). Sedgwick (1982), in a call for more constructive alliances, remarked upon shortcomings in the relationship between the wider labour movement and the politics of health and disability. Arguably, history shows that the interests of service users and the workforce do not always come together and service users could very well decline to join forces with staff they might blame for service failings (Wills and Simms, 2004).

Alternatively (as we have noted), there is the potential for service user and trade union objectives to coincide or interact, raising the potential for alliances between practitioners and service user or community activists. This would afford consideration of a number of associated themes and issues, including the nature of community and personhood, power dynamics within alliances, the need to establish more egalitarian relationships than those typically at stake in the provision of care and the rhetoric that sustains and promotes the action. Exploration of these themes offers a chance to address problems in previous relationships, especially where this has resulted in iniquitous power imbalances and stigmatised identities for service users.

3.8   Community Engaged Universities

Examples of community engagement involving universities can be found around the globe and the focus for this action can be equally varied. It may take the form of applied research projects, knowledge transfer, participatory projects, including action learning and action research, student and staff volunteering in the community, focused student study/research activity for community benefit, support for campaigns, direct involvement in community groups and movements, building alliances with professional and practitioner groups and associations, such as trade unions, forms of internationalism, widening access schemes for higher education, opening up university facilities for use by the community and facilitating the contribution of community groups and individuals to the range of university activity. The latter point best describes the involvement of service users and carers in teaching, research and other university business, but this particular focus can also create opportunities, or be a starting point, for many of the other forms of engagement listed. One way of looking at all this is to see it as a reciprocal sharing of resources between the university and its community; each having different forms of 'assets' and 'social capital'.

The universities, of course, also have significant material capital, and the mobilization of resources from the university into the community can be a tangible benefit of engaging with higher education institutions. Universities can help distribute material resources directly by allocating some of their own funds to community initiatives, or they can use their status, prestige and the skills of their academic workforce to lever in grant funding from elsewhere. Ball (2005) cites student learning as a vehicle for engagement, transacted through courses delivered by universities but focused on knowledge and skills relevant to effective community or civic engagement. Arguably, not all universities or academics involved in such processes will share a commitment to the social values or objectives of particular community projects, and the relationship may be paternalistic or, worse, parasitic. For example, their involvement prioritises self-serving objectives, such as research outputs and publications. Conversely, critically engaged academics will share common ground with community activists, sometimes in spite of relative institutional disinterest, and these relationships will more likely be sustained long after particular grant funded project work has been completed. In this sort of relationship, the products of engagement are shared, and though this might include academic outputs such as scholarly publications, these are not the be-all and end-all of the process.

The important characteristic of authentically participatory approaches is that research or learning is a two-way street in the spirit of Freire (1971). Participants are active in any study or enquiry, rather than passive objects or subjects of it. This relates to Barker and Cox's (2002) dissatisfaction with formal, academy-based, social movement studies and theorizing that is distant from the movements it seeks to study, especially removed from attachment to the movement's political goals. This 'contemplative' rather than action-orientated theory stops at finding explanations for phenomena, unlike the movement theory articulated by activists which always has political ends. These authors also wryly note how the growth in such university departments and subjects as social history, cultural studies and environmental studies has often been grounded in the work of 'organic intellectuals' from within movements. Various features of university culture are further impediments to crossing this divide, including career progression and tenure, research assessment exercises and pressure to secure funding. Despite these tensions, there are examples of critical academics who do manage to some extent to straddle the divide between academe and activism (Cox and Fominaya, 2009).

Critically engaged academics point out the value of the informal learning that takes place within participatory activity involving empowered citizens, service users or carers (Church, Bascia and Shragge, 2008). A number of examples of community initiatives that both inform and benefit from contributions from university academics are described in publications emanating from Toronto communities and staff at Ryerson University. These include innovative social enterprises and other collaborations involving mental health service users (Church, 1997, 2006a, 2006b, 2008a; Ignagni and Church, 2008) and research coalitions (Mental Health Recovery Study Group, 2009). Richter *et al.* (2003) describe how *Community Campus Partnerships for Health* has developed a policy highlighting the value of connecting community engagement with the traditional goals of universities – teaching, research and service. The aforementioned Toronto initiatives have generated numerous academic style publications, but also down to earth reports for community consumption and politicking, and a range of community events and exhibitions to render the work visible to the wider community (Voronka *et al.*, 2007; Church, 1995; Panitch *et al.*, 2008). Publication strategies also include attention to democratic and inclusive methods for attributing authorship in the spirit of creative commons (Church, 2008b; Mental Health Recovery Study Group, 2009).

These and other examples suggest that it is possible to create a kind of social enterprise that moves beyond modernist consumerist ideologies and towards genuine ideals of the creation of the common good, or even of common goods. Indeed, this turn of phrase slides easily into the concept of 'creative commons'. This approach to the knowledge economy sees intellectual property as a shared endeavour. From a classic ethical perspective, such an endeavour creates a virtuous cycle of beneficence, where shared knowledge provides a platform for the development of more shared knowledge, and society as a consequence can be improved for all, or, at least, for more. Declassified sharing of this nature stands in sharp contrast to the increasing commodification of knowledge within higher education institutes. In these settings, the production of intellectual property is highly valued and, indeed, required. In extreme instances, failure to produce exclusive intellectual property, through peer-reviewed publication, grant capture, or knowledge transfer consultancy, can be grounds for termination of employment.

This provides an obvious dilemma for social enterprise approaches to service user and carer engagement in universities. Even successful engagement schemes have to pay their way, by publication, and by earning external income through grant capture. This has two potentially maleficent consequences for those developing local projects. Firstly, time and energy are diverted away from the core business of supporting and engaging service users and carers. Secondly, those engaged in dissemination are forced to construct information about service users and carers in a way that meets the knowledge transfer standards of academia, but which may betray the values and principles of social enterprises that are seeking to work authentically in collaboration with their local community. Indeed, this debate has been current in the writing of this book, as notions of authorship and (thus) ownership of the knowledge product within it have been extensively discussed within the writing team.

There are alternatives to the academic commodification agenda. The concept of the creative commons may seem to be completely counter-productive in terms of increasingly commercial academia. However, there are classic cases that challenge this commonsense assumption. The most often quoted is that of the Canadian mining company, Goldcorp, which used the Internet, and the offer of a large cash prize, to marshal a mass response to the analysis of detailed geological survey data and indicate the most promising places to find gold deposits. The corporation eventually was pointed to around 90 productive sites, and over three billion dollars worth of gold was found, dwarfing the original prize amount of $575 000. The wholesale harnessing of public collaboration in pursuit of business objectives has become known as Crowdsourcing. The same ethos lies behind approaches to collective engagement in the design processes or inventing new technologies. Similarly, the term 'citizen science' has been applied to the mass participation of people with computers to analyse large amounts of data in the interests of mathematical or physical sciences for example. Such endeavours are made possible by the power of Internet technology, and Wikipedia is an obvious example of the potential afforded by large-scale cooperative enterprise using these media.

In terms of service user and carer engagement initiatives, dissemination of successful processes and procedures of engagement to the widest possible audience might be a good place to start. Normal academic routes, such as this book, or the Authenticity to Action conference referred to in Chapters 6 and 8, are one way of doing this (and see Chapter 6 for specific examples of tools and technique that could be used in other contexts). However, the opportunities afforded by the Internet, and by electronic media in general, offer almost limitless scope for such dissemination. Social networking sites like Facebook and YouTube, and highly networked systems like Twitter, provide rapid viral approaches to the dissemination of information and news. These are not only passively open access, but actively participatory. They offer the potential for the extreme opposite of tightly controlled guardianship of intellectual property rights and of exclusionary practices of knowledge sharing in contexts that can only be accessible to academic elites.

Ultimately, there is a happy medium to be struck between a highly regulated quality control approach to dissemination and social marketing based on a particular kind of authoritative knowledge, and a completely deregulated system, where any bundle of information is as valid and as valuable as any other. To get this balance right, the emotional intelligence that is a component of much service user and carer input needs to be valued alongside 'normal science' scientific knowledge (Chapter 5). Indeed, for a health and social care audience, emotional intelligence might be the vital missing element that service users and carers can provide. Participatory open access examples, such as Dipex, offer information created by service users and carers that is carefully constructed and which acknowledges the effort and creativity of those who are involved. These examples stand for many others, as the possibilities in this area multiply exponentially. If the creative commons movement can strike a balance between acknowledging the intellectual and emotional input of service users and carers and the academics who work with them, and the open access methods supported by new technologies, it is possible that the demands of universities and of authentic service user engagement can both be met.

Community engagement initiatives involving universities or academic staff can avoid paternalism and become truly participatory and radical. Calderon (2004: 91) concludes that they can be:

> a practical means for promoting positive social relations by building bridges between students, faculty and community participants from diverse backgrounds; [moving] beyond top-down charity and project development models to models based on collaborative action for social change.

There is wide-ranging literature, with some key foci in social geography and the politics of social movements, that critiques and help us make sense of the relationships between universities and their local communities. A feature of this literature is theory that brings identity issues to the fore and also engages with the expression of purpose as a form of discourse. With reference to a different context, it has been argued that trade unions need to be equally concerned with their community relations as they are with the instrumentalism of workplace objectives, and that this may be achieved by reinventing themselves as discourse organizations. For those academics interested in the potential for improving the relationships between universities and communities, one might equally suggest that the university ought to be seen as a discourse organization. This imperative would pose a number of questions. What are universities actually for? What is the story being told? How is the university presenting itself? How authentic or reciprocal is the attachment to the community?

The response of a university as a discourse organization would be to get its message out in a clear and understandable way. Hopefully, this would be a message reflecting a strong community-orientated mission. In this context, community relationships are paramount and discourse is about 'doing' as much as theorizing. Involvement in collaborative university community engagement projects and wider community politics opens up a space for reflecting upon the nature of academic and community identities. In a context of increasing commercialization of universities, retraction of staffing and course provision, more profound existential issues arise, including those which question the very purpose of the university and its role in a community.

3.9   Alienation and Redemption

Wrapped up with questions about the role and purpose of universities are important considerations for the identity of those staff who work within them. These can be seen to be similar to crises of identity which face practitioners working in health and social care services. Arguably, all of these staff, regardless of setting, can experience dissonance between how they would prefer to see themselves (and have others see them) and how this might be compromised by the ways in which their work is organised beyond their control (McKeown and Spandler, 2006). Such staff would clearly experience alienation in their job roles. Arguably, critically engaged practitioners and academics would be, at one and the same time, most sensitive to experience this, but also best placed to redeem their situation through the work fulfilment that comes from authentic alliances with service users and communities. Arenas of health and social care practice are an opportune place to explore this notion of alienation, before turning to the possibilities afforded within universities concerned with health and social care.

Despite the emphasis in classical Marxism, alienation and its flip-side, work as self-realization, is a neglected concept in analyses of health and medicine, even amongst Marxist commentators on the subject (Yuill, 2005). One exception is Cohen (1995), who pointed out that a Marxist notion of alienation reflects people's attachment to personal autonomy and self-ownership, concepts usually appropriated by libertarians rather than socialists. For Cohen, the privatization of property is a form of restriction of people's freedoms to use things owned by others; this perspective challenged the view of right-wing thinkers that demands for equality alone posed a threat to liberty.

Yuill (2005) has attempted to resurrect interest in alienation within medical sociology, and draws attention to the centrality in Marx's thought of notions of embodiment and emotions, and how these are distorted by labour under capitalism leading to poor health outcomes. Yuill (2005) makes the connection in this context with more modern theories of emotional labour. Marx was interested in people as social beings, and it is their social relationships that shape their consciousness (McLennan, 1977). Marx rejects the idea of an unvarying human nature, seeing the potential for completely altruistic relationships checked by prevailing social and economic conditions (Coates, 1990).

'Species being' is only fully realised in communistic society, with people maximizing creativity and cooperation amongst their fellows. It is the way in which work is organised and controlled that exploits and alienates workers. Marx is highly critical of this state of affairs under capitalism, not just because it is exploitative and unfair but also because this damages our development as human beings (Porter, 1998). Health and social care jobs can be rewarding and satisfying but, arguably, various developments in the organization of modern services render them implicitly alienating, perhaps accounting for some of the evidence relating to workplace stress and burnout.

This can happen on two levels. First, the application of technologies of care and treatment is accomplished at the expense of staff autonomy and control over working practices. Individual workers experience alienation because the organization of their work divorces them from a stake in all aspects of the job, especially the finished 'product'. Unrewarding work is most likely to resemble the sort of task allocation seen on factory production lines, and the most rewarding work is akin to pre-industrial craftwork or newer visions of flexible specialization. Task allocation and tendency to minimise practitioner autonomy are exaggerated by the dominance of narrow medicalised conceptual frameworks and the creeping introduction of managerialism and marketization. Second, is the alienation that arises when one's self-image and role aspirations are at odds with experiences of work. Marx identified the notion of 'species being' to describe the alienation occurring when an individual's need to work and contribute to the welfare of fellows and family members is undermined. People become alienated from themselves, from one another and also from their social world, their community.

In this sense, the experience of work unsettles people's very sense of self and identity. Arguably, practitioners would prefer to think of themselves as caring individuals making positive contributions to the lives of service users. However, the actuality of these roles commonly threatens this idealised sense of identity, with practitioners often finding themselves in conflictual relationships with service users. The effect of this is to engender service user dissatisfaction with services, associated with their experience of individual workers. These practitioners are placed in the position of wishing to make a positive impact in people's lives and for that to be appreciated, whereas the actual experience is to be perceived negatively and feel unappreciated.

The organization of health and social care work has been analyzed by various commentators. It has been argued that Braverman's critique of industrialised production, division of labour and degraded experience of work was equally applicable to human services occupations (Doyal, 1979; Carey, 2009). The visible fragmentation and specialization of the labour process is not even primarily concerned with the most efficient organization of work, rather it is a means by which control is exerted over the workforce.

Successive reorganizations and market-orientated reforms of the UK National Health Service have operated to progressively exacerbate tendencies towards fragmentation of tasks and control over practitioners' work (McKeown, 1995; Towers, 1996). Similarly, research has highlighted workers' discomfort with prevailing ideologies with Bolton (2001: 94) finding nurses 'alienated from the concept of treating patients as customers'. Alternative models for organizing the labour process, offering workers involvement in all stages, from planning to implementation, might be the antidote to alienating features and actually be more productive (Wood, 1989). Piore and Sable (1984) describe a system of flexible specialization modelled upon the re-emergence of craft skills, optimizing worker autonomy and flattening out hierarchies. Such approaches correspond with an ideal-typical conceptualization of nurses' work, organised around the craft of caring, maximizing autonomy and continuity in caring relationships (McKeown, 1995).

Cooperative, non-hierarchical team-working might also reduce feelings of alienation. However, if team structure reproduces hierarchies and status differentials in the division of labour, then it can actually exacerbate alienation (Cott, 1998). This is especially the case amongst lower grades of staff with less resources and chances to alter their status, but who are key to implementing decisions made by higher status professionals. Cott (1998) notes that alienation arising from the social structure for staff in hospitals is not news. This is greater amongst staff experiencing routinised, mechanical conceptions of their work (Coser, 1963) and where rigid, impersonal structures of authority prevail (Pearlin, 1962). The dominant ideology of biological psychiatry in mental health services, for example, allied with prominent discourses of risk and governance, can exacerbate the extent to which workers feel subject to control. Various commentators have drawn upon a notion of emotional labour (Jones, 1994; James, 1992; Bolton, 2001) to highlight stress associated with the sort of intimacy and interpersonal relationships central to the work of health and social care practitioners. James (1992) suggests that routinization of work undermines models of individualised care that more thoroughly engage with these emotional aspects.

It is also worth noting the commodification and reification of relationships inherent in some of the prevailing language in caring services. Relationships become 'packages' of care and support becomes 'input'. Certain health and social care professionals are increasingly given the role of promoting social inclusion and social capital. While this offers some opportunities for developing genuine social relationships and challenging exclusionary social practices, the language of social inclusion 'commodifies our relations with ourselves, as we treat ourselves and our capacities as marketable commodities, and does the same with social relationships' (Levitas, 2004: 10). Workers are increasingly alienated from the 'product' of their labour (the service users themselves and their experiences of ill health or social needs) as well as being denied access to fulfilling relationships and influence over the wider context of people's lives. In this sense, workers can increasingly be seen as alienated from 'species being' (i.e. genuine human and social relationships).

Many staff experience alienation, and at least part of this relates to ways in which the organization of work blocks opportunities to engage in meaningful alliances with service users. The fact that service users have emerged as a social movement, largely dissatisfied in their engagement with services, suggests that the experience of health and social care services can be alienating for all concerned, staff and service users. This leads us to concur with Sedgwick's plea for a grass roots collectivised approach to services, unifying the needs of users, workers and carers (Sedgwick, 1982). There is potential for service user activism to be implicitly life-affirming and promote well-being (Fanon, 1967). Staff connections and alliances with the growing service user movement may offer similar rewards. The possibility of staff collective organizations forging links with community activism and newer social movements possibly offers a glimmer of opportunity for the reinvigoration of some aspects of the traditional labour movement.

Individual funding schemes such as direct payments are becoming more and more popular, especially in social care, and will possibly even be extended to health care in the United Kingdom. Such mechanisms give service users money in lieu of services, so they can arrange and purchase their own support to meet their assessed care needs. This may offer service users the opportunity to develop their own individually tailored responses to their needs. However, there are still some unresolved questions and suspicions that these will entail further rationing of care and be associated with unwelcome privatization and curtailing of community resources for those who still wish to use directly provided services (Spandler, 2004). In some ways individual funding mechanisms offer opportunities for new and innovative partnerships between service users, carers and workers through various mechanisms, such as advance directives and new working contracts (Spandler and Heslop 2007). Radical developments could include politicised alternatives and self-help organizations, such as networks of people who hear voices, experience paranoia or self-harm in the mental health field (Jacobson and Zavos, 2007; Cresswell, 2005). On the other hand, there are concerns that direct payments could result in further avenues for alienation if workers (or personal assistants) are isolated, unsupported and un-unionised. Ultimately, tipping the balance in favour of greater collaboration will depend, at least in part, on the strength of independent service user and carer organizations and their ability to develop links with workers and trade unions (Cresswell and Spandler, 2009).

It would be naive to recommend a simple notion of 'user involvement' as a 'non-alienating' remedy for all perceived ills. Partly because of the way this term has been so co-opted and incorporated into top-down managerial and policy initiatives, partly because of conflicting ideologies at stake in different versions of involvement and activism, such as in the tensions between new and old social movements. There is ample room to concern ourselves with more sophisticated understandings of this territory and disaggregate the notion of user involvement and alliances to arrive at those elements and contexts with the most potential for radical ends. This might boil down to a focus on mutual relations of care, support and action, resonant with Delanty's concept of personalism. Such an approach might open up links between progressive health and social care work and empowered service users and carers active in social movements or other forms of community and civic engagement. This might occur in forms of collective action or consciousness-raising between workers and users. There might also be opportunities for all concerned to confront stigmatizing constructions of difference, adopting alternative notions of self and identity, framed around common humanity and connectedness rather than pathology.

In an example of prefiguration in action, Crossley (1999b) has outlined the idea of 'working utopias' as mini-realizations of imagined changes desired by the user movement. They are 'working sites' of alternative practices or 'laboratories of experience' which bring together radical practitioners, activists and theorists, providing common reference points as well as actual meeting places for the generation of radical ideas which are important in reproducing social movement knowledge and activism.

Community engagement activities for universities involve partnerships and alliances between university staff and individuals and self-organised groups in the local community from a range of different user and carer perspectives. The research findings of the Comensus project (Chapter 9) reflect wider observations regarding new social movements with strong themes around activism, common purpose, altruism, friendships, mutuality and solidarity in the emerging relationships. The university staff with a health or social care practice background report opportunities for more fulfilling and rewarding relationships than were necessarily available to them as practitioners (Chapter 8). This might reflect the relative ease in establishing egalitarian and mutually empowering connections where the issue of direct care delivery is not immediately at stake. Whatever the reasons might prove to be, it is clear that *different* sorts of relationships *are* possible when efforts are made towards building alliances in different contexts.

In the UK mental health survivors movement, for example, a largely user-led initiative to preserve the movement's history is supported by a network of roughly a hundred members, the Survivor's History Group. Within this grouping, a number of academic supporters who are not personally part of the survivors' movement have made notable contributions, including writing portions of the history of the movement (Campbell and Roberts, 2009). Some of this history includes moments in time where staff and service user alliances were important (Spandler, 2006). Arguably, the growth and autonomy of the user movement perhaps means that it is no longer dependent on such alliances to flourish. Yet the very potential for alliance raises the prospect of interesting dimensions of solidarity that challenge negative, stigmatised constructions of difference.

The delicate distinction between 'workers' and 'service users' is always clouded by the experience of distress endemic in modern society. Indeed, Sedgwick drew attention to a passionate concern with what he regarded as the great seriousness and specificity of mental illnesses which can debilitate the working classes, including, and especially, mental health workers and political militants of various progressive causes (Lukes, 1984). Radical strategies must increase the possibilities of greater self-determination addressing the needs of recipients *and* workers.

Highlighting issues of alienation or fulfilment in professional encounters is more than just an abstract or academic exercise. Such matters are worthy of consideration, especially in the preparation of future generations of practitioners. These individuals will go on to occupy professional roles, affording them opportunities to become involved in trade unions and connect with service user and carer organizations. Policy developments like personal budgets present some tricky challenges to the notion of alliance in encounters with service users, further reinforcing the need for service users, carers and workers, including personal assistants, to come together in learning. Arguably, prior reflection on the value of personal, therapeutic and political alliances is a crucial part of a rounded professional education.

The key to undermining alienating relationships is the transformation of the social structures and cultures sustaining them. The social history of health and social care suggests a strong vein of radicalism is available to practitioners, if at times the expression of this is muted or constrained. One possible route to more rewarding and less alienating care practices is through alliances on various levels with service users, organised service user groups and community activists. Institutional responses can hazard potential beneficial effects through processes of co-option and incorporation. Our tentative conclusion is that there is a need for practitioners and academics to be in touch with and connected to broader social movements, to nourish their alliances and facilitate progressive ways of working beyond narrow notions of user 'involvement' and 'consultation'. The idea of 'critically engaged' academics and academies is an interesting starting point for pursuing this in a university/community context, heralding the possibility of working towards universities as 'mini-utopias' of progressive and prefigurative practices, and hopefully greater fulfilment in role and positive sense of identity for the staff who work in them.

4 Research and Evaluation of Service Users' and Carers' Involvement in Health Professional Education

Janice L. Hanson and Beth A. Lown

An ongoing interest in and abiding respect for people with special healthcare needs have motivated and shaped my career, firstly in special education, then in medical education. As a teacher, I asked my students and their families about their lives and needs, struggles and triumphs, always learning from their stories. Variously, they told me about experiences with doctors and nurses, therapists and social workers, in hospitals, clinics, offices and home therapy programmes. I quickly learned that those of us who were trying to help would do a much better job if we learned to listen carefully, and to shape our programmes, interventions, care and systems according to the insights we gained from the people living with needs that required health care or special education. By the time I began to plan my doctoral dissertation in 1980, it was clear to me that I would structure my research and work to build ways to learn systematically from people living with disabilities and health conditions. And so my journey has continued – from special education to healthcare, with parents and patients as advisors, to medical education and beyond, always seeking ways to listen and to shape the systems of care within which I worked according to the insights I gained. Much later, in 1994, we faced serious and chronic health challenges in my own family, as my husband encountered a sequence of stunning intrusions in his previously healthy life. I found myself in the role of carer and tenacious advocate as we negotiated the stormy waters of the crises, and then as we learned to live our lives in circumstances forever changed by these events. I had already known that the 'patients and their families' were my colleagues and teachers. These personal experiences have served to anchor in my soul the importance of working together as we care, give, teach, learn and make a difference through education, always integrating stories and wisdom from the lives of those we walk alongside. (Janice Hanson, Uniformed Services University of the Health Sciences, Bethesda, Maryland, USA)

My thoughts, emotions and orientation towards social activism were shaped during an era of significant social upheaval in the United States. Those were the days of the civil rights, women's, and students' movements and they instilled in me a sense of collaboration and responsibility for co-creating a more equitable, participatory democracy. I chose a life of service through the practice of primary care medicine. When I entered medical school, there were few role models from whom to learn ways of being with others that honoured their whole life contexts and experiences. But I knew that, as much as I needed to learn the science of medicine, so too did I need to learn from patients about the ways of their bodies, hearts, souls and minds. Only by listening to their stories, hearing their personal wisdom and integrating this with my own would I be able to act as a partner in fostering health and managing illness. No doubt, my personal role as a carer for family members with mental health issues deepened my commitment to supporting and helping others find their own ways to health. Now I do more teaching than doctoring, but my commitment to learning and helping others learn how healthcare relationships can serve as a source of caring, support, and shared wisdom has not waned. I hold this sense of purpose deeply and carefully. (Beth Lown, Mount Auburn Hospital, Cambridge, Massachusetts, USA)

4.1 Introduction

At Mount Auburn Hospital in Cambridge, Massachusetts, physicians in post-graduate training in radiology were uncomfortable speaking directly with women in the mammography suite about their abnormal mammograms. Not all of the staff radiologists enjoyed that assignment either. The rapid pace and volume of patient throughput created challenges. Perhaps more importantly, many of the physicians in training simply did not know how to respond when a person burst into tears, appeared fearful or questioned the uncertainty inevitably inherent in radiologic interpretation. Furthermore, radiologists, unlike primary care physicians or general practitioners, have no previous or ongoing relationships upon which to build such difficult conversations. Nevertheless, the hospital was committed to providing women with immediate information about their diagnostic mammograms in order to meet women's preferences (Levin *et al.*, 2000; Raza *et al.*, 2001), potentially reduce their anxiety and enhance follow up (Barton *et al.*, 2004). In response, the training programme involved women who had survived breast cancer in designing and teaching a communications curriculum, and in providing feedback and evaluation of the trainees' communication skills (Lown, Sasson and Hinrichs, 2008).

Educators at the Uniformed Services University of the Health Sciences in Bethesda, Maryland, created a programme to teach medical students during their family medicine clerkship about advocating for individuals and families in healthcare systems and communities, and how to plan healthcare management grounded in the context of people's lives. People with complex or chronic health conditions worked with faculty to develop a new teaching programme about health and disease in life context, and patients, parents and medical school faculty began co-teaching a workshop about advocacy. Service users and family members also worked with the faculty to write standardised cases to assess whether students had acquired the communication skills, understanding of users perspectives, and knowledge of healthcare and community resources needed to address the needs of individuals and families (Hanson and Randall, 2007a).

Faculty in schools of medicine, psychology, social work and other health professional education programmes have developed curricular activities like these at many universities, hospitals and other community settings around the world. The first challenge is to get the programmes started. Hand in hand with that challenge comes the next: involving service users and families in designing and implementing evaluation of these innovative programmes, and designing research to determine whether the practices, insights and outcomes of these health professional education programmes will transfer or generalise more widely. This chapter describes evaluation and research methods for health professional education programmes in which service users, carers and other faculty teach and learn together. The chapter also references examples of efforts by those who have applied these methods, and discusses collaboration of service users, carers and other faculty in setting a research agenda, designing systematic research and evaluation processes, gathering data and interpreting results.

Recent reviews of the literature provide numerous papers and valuable descriptions of the variety of ways in which service users and carers have been involved in health professional education (Spencer *et al.*, 2000; Wykurz and Kelly, 2002; Jha *et al.*, 2009a). The spectrum of reported involvement of service users and carers varies in the duration of contact with learners, the degree of service user or carer autonomy during teaching encounters, the amount of preparation for teaching, the amount of service user and carer involvement in planning and evaluation, and the degree of institutional commitment to their involvement (Tew, Gell and Foster, 2004; Towle and Goldolphin, 2008). Examples of involvement include: eliciting service user or carer input with regard to training content (Rudman, 1996; Flanagan, 1999; Randall and Hanson, 2000; Sawley, 2002); developing learning materials (Coupland, Davis and Gregory, 2001; Hanson and Randall, 2007b); providing feedback on professional skills through questionnaires (Greco, Brownlea and Mcgovern, 2001); and interacting with learners as teachers and as evaluators (Branch *et al.*, 1999; Hendry, Schrieber and Bryce, 1999; Davidson *et al.*, 2001; Haq, Fuller and Dacre, 2006). The teaching and evaluation have most frequently been in the area of communication and physical examination skills. These papers provide the reader with insight about how the authors framed the results of their educational programmes, and to some extent they provide examples of evaluation and approaches to educational research. The majority of these papers, however, describe programmes with little focus on evaluation or research. Those that do address evaluation generally focus on the evaluation of participants' reactions to and satisfaction with the programmes, and do not attempt to measure more concrete or long-term outcomes.

Programme evaluation is essential if goals include the development and continuous improvement of effective educational models that involve service users and carers. Educational research is essential if goals include the development of transferable or generaliseable insights and theories about what elements of these programmes foster intended goals and facilitate behavioural and institutional change. When developing a new programme for health professional education or evaluating how well a programme works in a particular setting, it is helpful to think about different levels of outcomes. These levels may include changes in learner knowledge, skills, attitudes and behaviour, and impact on a healthcare setting or community. When seeking to discover knowledge that may generalise or transfer to other educational settings, in addition to thinking about levels of educational outcomes, careful choice of a research design is important.

When planning a programme evaluation, Kirkpatrick's four levels of evaluation provide a helpful framework (Kirkpatrick, 1998). Level 1 is reaction (how well learners liked the programme), level 2 is learning (what knowledge or skills were learned), level 3 is behaviour (what changes in behaviour or skills resulted from the programme) and level 4 is results (what tangible outcomes resulted from the programme). In the literature, most of the papers about educational programmes that include service users and carers describe what the programmes do, what educational and administrative processes they have established and how teachers and learners react to them. Few, however, assess Kirkpatrick's higher levels of evaluation, such as changes in attitudes and actual behaviours in clinical settings, or the impact of programmes on educational institutions and on the communities in which participants live. Descriptions of service user and carer involvement in health professional education have served a useful purpose in the literature, helping to stimulate the development of innovative programmes that involve patients and families in co-teaching and shaping the form of health professional education. The challenge that remains, however, is to move beyond description and evaluation of process to that of outcomes and meaningful impact, facilitating the development of theories and models about learning in programmes that involve service users and carers and providing insights about behavioural and social change upon which an international community of educators can build.

Educational research on service user and carer involvement in health professional education, like social and behavioural science research in general, is hard to do well. Most educational research never makes it from projects to published papers, and most published papers in education never appear in the citations of papers by other authors (Kline, 2009). There are probably many reasons for this, including limited resources and the difficulties inherent in doing robust educational research. Educational research in a contrived setting that controls variables for precise measurement would have little relevance in the real world, and educational research in the real world involves multiple variables and complicated context. Nonetheless, programme evaluators and educational researchers who create guiding questions that focus on learning outcomes and the impact of educational programmes will more likely make a difference with the work they do. This chapter will address some of the challenges of both programme evaluation and medical education research by suggesting evaluation and research outcomes that make a difference when involving service users and carers in health professional education, and by describing research designs and methods that will help educators address meaningful questions with sound design and a bit of creativity as well.

4.2   At the Start: Clarify Your Vision and Choose a Question to Address and an Outcome that Makes a Difference

What drives us to build a new educational programme, to share our own health-care experiences in a teaching setting, or to involve service users and families in the teaching we do? How do we establish a vision and a set of goals? Our vision and goals come from a sense in our hearts and minds that there is a gap between our values and our practice, between what we believe in our hearts will make healthcare work well and what we experience in the healthcare setting, or between our values and educational outcomes. Research and evaluation questions begin to emerge when we see something that is not right, discern how to address it, and then decide how to determine whether we have made any progress. For example, we might decide that our core values are compassion, kindness, relationships, equality, respect and justice. If we then see programmes, behaviours, learning and outcomes that contradict this set of values, we decide to take action. Action includes writing a good question that addresses the gap between our values and the practices and outcomes of educational programmes for health professionals.

This chapter is a call to action, a call to examine gaps between personal experience of service user and carer involvement in health professional education and a particular vision of ideal involvement, or between outcomes of educational programmes and goals for learners. If a gap is seen, the optimum response is to write a question about it, design a plan to initiate change, and then figure out how to evaluate the impact of the change. For example:

At Mount Auburn Hospital, the questions that guided the project to address the educational need of the radiology residents were these: What should effective, person-centred communication look and sound like? Who should decide what constitutes 'best communication practices' in this discipline? Their educational research group (a radiologist, a patient-trainer and educator, and an internal medicine physician with communication expertise) began by agreeing upon the fundamental belief that best communication practices should be collaboratively co-constructed and co-taught with women who had received the news of an abnormal mammogram working with the physicians, educators and learners throughout the project. They initiated their research by asking service users who had undergone diagnostic mammograms, experienced radiologists, and radiology residents in training to help build an understanding of their experiences.

As a second example:

At the Uniformed Services University, service users and families working in the educational programme emphasised the importance of doctors' communication with them, and the importance of planning healthcare in a way that helped them live their lives at home, work and school. When the family medicine clerkship developed a new workshop for medical students, the family medicine faculty worked with the service user and family faculty to write four standardised service user cases that assessed the medical students' skills in basic communication and in building relationships, efforts to plan with service users and referral to healthcare and community resources that could help address a person's health problem.

4.3   Service Users, Carers and Other Faculty Work as Partners in Research and Evaluation of Health Professional Education

We may initially find ourselves working together because this supports our values or implements public policies or grant proposal requirements that promote involvement of service users and carers. For example, the National Health Service Constitution in the United Kingdom specifies that service users and carers will participate in health professional education and in planning and implementing healthcare research (DH, 2009b). In the United States, the National Institutes of Health requires that all proposals for Clinical and Translational Science awards, which fund multimillion dollar, multidisciplinary healthcare research and education projects, include specific and meaningful plans for community engagement in the planning and implementation of the projects (NIH, 2009). It becomes clear, however, that we can design programmes that promote health and heal illness only if we consider the perspectives and lived experiences of those most affected by such programmes. Identifying the most important questions and truly meaningful outcomes requires integrating the perspectives of those who live most closely with the results of teaching and the systems of care, as well as the perspectives of professional educators and researchers. Systematic evaluation and research help educators translate these ideas into practice and measure the outcomes.

Service users, carers and other faculty can play important roles in all phases of research and evaluation, from planning through data collection and its interpretation. Some may bring their perspectives and priorities to decisions about the focus of research and evaluation, choices about design and methods and approaches to analysis and interpretation, while others may bring technical expertise about teaching, research and evaluation methods. The goal of this work, however, is to collaborate fully in decision making and the activities of the research effort, from the beginning and in each thing we do. Some of the roles that service users and carers and other faculty can fill together in research and evaluation include the following:

1. Look at the domains of potential outcomes and decide what areas of impact best fit a particular educational programme, organization and community.
2. Write questions and goals for research agendas.
3. Write specific goals and objectives for a particular research or evaluation project.

4. Critique a set of evaluation or research goals or questions in terms of comprehensiveness and importance, integrating different perspectives in the critique.
5. Critique a draft of a research or evaluation project design in relation to whether the procedures convey respect for participants.
6. Write questions for interviews, focus groups and surveys.
7. Create easily understood instructions for research participants.
8. Write informed consent documents that incorporate service users and carers' perspectives of potential risks of participation, and that are short yet complete, straightforward, and understandable.
9. Define variables for educational intervention studies.
10. Participate as interviewers, observers and note-takers.
11. Serve as research participants in interviews, focus groups, surveys and other measures of outcomes.
12. Interpret research results.
13. Prepare and present research results for service users, families, community groups, educators, policy and programme planners and leaders, ensuring that differing perspectives are appropriately represented.

Each member of the team brings unique and important perspectives and contributions, and the evaluation effort is richer when it represents this diversity. Individuals and health professional institutions may, however, vary greatly in their motivation, ability and the resources available to incorporate the views of service users and carers in educational planning, education and research, and service users and carers may distrust efforts to do so. Efforts to introduce changes to long-established approaches to these tasks can be daunting. We may find ourselves tempted to lessen the magnitude of these efforts by seeking solutions that inadvertently limit access to participation or representation of important perspectives. For example, we may seek the participation of service users and carers who also have formal expertise in research and evaluation, or educators and researchers who feel they can adequately represent the perspectives of service users and carers. With perseverance, however, service users, carers and other faculty can deepen their understanding of the experience of illness as well as of evaluation and research methods as they work together over time.

4.4 Domains of Outcomes of Service User and Family Involvement in Health Professional Education

Pursuing goals for education that incorporate service users and carers in meaningful ways requires turning attention toward the domains in which we collectively hope to have an impact. Who or what do we hope to affect with an educational programme? In other words, who is the target audience for change? We may want to target several audiences within education, service user and carer communities.

We may hope for broader organizational change, such as a change in the culture of an educational institution, a change in the healthcare system where service users and families receive care, or a change in the communities in which people live and work. We may hope to contribute to national or international literature about health professional education.

Another way to think about the impact we hope to evaluate or study is to consider our desired outcomes in terms of the levels of programme evaluation described by Kirkpatrick and outlined previously (Kirkpatrick, 1998). Level one is the participants' reactions to the educational programme – for example their satisfaction, degree of participation, or sense of satisfaction about their learning (for students), or satisfaction with their contribution to learning (for service users, carers and other faculty). Level two encompasses the learning that results from the programme, such as the knowledge and attitudes acquired by students, new insights and attitudes acquired by healthcare providers who serve as faculty, or the new skills or insights acquired by the service users and carers who also teach. Level three includes changes in behaviour. What do the students do differently in their clinical practice settings? What do the service users and carers who serve as educators do differently when they seek their own healthcare, or when they work or teach in their communities? What do faculty members do differently when teaching? Finally, level four comprises various kinds of impact on organizations or communities. What changes occurred in the culture of an educational setting, a hospital or clinic, or the culture of the communities in which students, service users or carers and other faculty members live and work?

Table 4.1 summarises these domains of impact for evaluation or research study outcomes, and provides some examples of the outcomes that might be described or measured. When choosing outcomes for evaluation or research, the key is to focus on outcomes that describe a meaningful result of the involvement of service users or carers in an educational programme. In some fields of research, the 'gold standard' is a randomised controlled trial. In educational evaluation or research that is embedded in the context of a social or educational setting, however, a randomised controlled trial may not provide the best way to determine the outcomes of the work. Evaluation and research in such settings is best designed by determining the outcomes that are meaningful to participants, and then choosing (from the wide array of research and evaluation strategies described in the sections below) the approach that best assesses these outcomes.

4.5 Research and Evaluation Design

Research and evaluation designs provide a way to plan a systematic approach to studying meaningful outcomes of education. The designs provide the basic plan, and methods (discussed in the next section) provide ways to implement the plan. A systematic plan and use of rigorous methods helps educators gather information that will best aid in decisions about how to improve teaching. A systematic

Table 4.1 Outcomes for research and evaluation.

Domain of outcomes	Kirkpatrick level	Sample questions for evaluation or research	Sample studies reported in the literature
Process evaluation	Not addressed by Kirkpatrick levels. Addresses the questions, 'Did we do what we set out to do? How did we do it? How did we plan? How many people participated? Which groups and perspectives did they represent?'	In what roles did service users and carers participate in our planning process and teaching? What was the process by which programme components were developed and implemented? Which programme components did we change or complete?	The UCLan community engagement and service user support (Comensus) project: Valuing authenticity, making space for emergence (Downe et al., 2007).
Satisfaction and other responses of participants	Level one (impact on reactions)	How do students and faculty react to the educational programmes involving service users as teachers? How did service users and carers react to participating as teachers in an educational programme for students? What is teacher or learner satisfaction with the programme?	What educators and students really think about using patients as teachers in medical education: A qualitative study (Jha et al., 2009b). Patients as teachers: A qualitative study of patients' views on their role in a community-based undergraduate project (Stacy and Spencer, 1999).
Impact of service users and carers on the learners a. Attitudes b. Practice behaviour, skills c. Knowledge, insight, understanding	Level two (impact on learning) Level three (impact on behaviour)	How did learners' attitudes about service user and family participation in decisions change during and after the educational programme? Can an educational intervention by trained persons with arthritis have a positive impact on retention of information, confidence and examination skills of medical students? How does the impact of lay teaching associates on students' physical examination skills compare with the impact of faculty?	Mutual influence in shared decision making; a collaborative study of patients and physicians (Lown, Hanson and Clark, 2009). Positive impact of an intervention by arthritis educators on retention of information, confidence and examination skills of medical students (Branch and Lipsky, 1998). Teaching foundational physical examination skills: study results comparing lay teaching associates and physician instructors (Barley et al., 2006).

		What skills for shared decision making did learners apply during supervised clinical learning experiences? What knowledge did learners gain about 'the context of a patient's life'?	
Impact of involvement in health professional education on service users and carers a. Attitudes b. Skills, behaviours in healthcare, as educators, in the community c. Knowledge, insight, understanding	Level two (impact on learning) Level three (impact on behaviour)	After participating in teaching, how did the confidence of service users and carers change regarding raising questions with their own healthcare providers? What teaching skills did service users and carers gain after participating in our educational programme? Does participation in health professional education affect the health and quality of life of service users and carers who teach? What knowledge did service user and family teachers gain about how to navigate the healthcare system?	'A stronger and clearer perception of self.' Women's experience of being professional patients in teaching the pelvic examination: a qualitative study (Siwe, Wijma and Bertero, 2006). What happens to patients who teach? (Gecht, 2000).
Impact of service users' and carers' involvement on the 'culture' of the school, the learning environment, or the institution	Level four (impact on organizations)	How has the involvement of service users and families as teachers changed the content of our curriculum? How did student descriptions of the learning environment change before and after the programme involved service users and families as teachers? How has the culture of our institution changed since the change in our educational programme?	Advancing a partnership: Patients, families and medical educators (Hanson and Randall, 2007a). We could find no examples of change in health professional learning environments or institutional culture associated with involvement of service users or carers. However, 'Enhancing the informal curriculum of a medical school: A case study in organizational culture change' provides an example of culture change in an academic health centre (Cottingham et al., 2008).

(Continued)

Table 4.1 (*Continued*)

Domain of outcomes	Kirkpatrick level	Sample questions for evaluation or research	Sample studies reported in the literature
Impact of service users' and carers' involvement in health professional education on healthcare a. How care is delivered (healthcare system practices) b. Health outcomes (including benchmarks and tracked quality measures used in quality assurance programmes)	Level four (impact on organizations)	How has our discharge planning process changed to more fully include service users and families in discharge planning decisions? Since our educational programme, what changes have occurred regarding service users successful follow-through on agreed-upon medication plans? What has the impact of our educational intervention been on the need for service user re-hospitalization?	The care transitions intervention: Results of a randomised controlled trial (Coleman *et al.*, 2006).
Impact of involvement on communities through a. Service users and families b. Faculty c. Advocacy groups d. Learners	Level four (impact on organizations) and beyond	What new educational efforts about healthcare have service users and carers started or enhanced after participating in our educational programmes? How have community-based patient advocacy groups changed through participation by faculty, service users, carers, or learners who completed our educational programme? How have community-based service users and carers participated in the oversight and implementation of new curricula in ambulatory settings? Does the degree of service user and carer involvement correlated with positive educational outcomes?	'No fear' curricular change: Monitoring curricular change in the W. K. Kellogg Foundation's National Initiative on Community Partnerships and Health Professions Education (Bland *et al.*, 2000). Leadership behaviours for successful university–community collaborations to change curricula (Bland *et al.*, 1999).

approach and rigorous research also build credibility for educational work. Providing good education for health professionals, and integrating the insight and expertise of service users and carers, is important work that warrants care, attention and resources for systematic evaluation and study, as well as high quality teaching.

Traditionally, research has sought the discovery of new information. More recently, several influential thinkers, for example Ernest Boyer and Charles Glassick (Boyer, 1990; Glassick, 2000a; Glassick, 2000b; Simpson *et al.*, 2007), have promoted a broader view of scholarship to include not only the discovery of new information but also systematic approaches to the development and evaluation of teaching and the application of insights and information discovered by others. Descriptions of the scholarship of teaching and the scholarship of application provide a framework for approaching the evaluation of teaching and the application of curricular strategies in a particular educational setting. The results can answer local questions, which is important, and may be applicable to other programmes with similar goals, values and innovations. The criteria for good scholarship can help planners organise a systematic, thoughtful approach. The criteria include the following (Tewksbury *et al.*, 2009):

a. **Clear goals.** Is the basic purpose of the project well defined? Do the objectives of the project address a problem of importance or consequence? Are the objectives realistic and achievable?
b. **Adequate preparation.** Does the educator show an understanding of existing scholarship relevant to the project? Does the project benefit from the educator's own skills and expertise? Are resources used appropriately to advance the project?
c. **Appropriate methods.** Are the methods chosen and applied appropriate for the project? Are the methods modified as necessary?
d. **Significant results.** What is the evidence of the success of the project? Are the goals achieved? Do the results contribute notably to the field in a manner that invites further explorations?
e. **Effective presentation.** Is the presentation of the project in a suitable format? Is it well organised and clear? Will it reach the intended audience?
f. **Reflective critique.** Has the educator thoughtfully assessed the project using his/her own perceptions as well as the critique from others to refine, enhance or expand the original concept?

It is important to determine whether the intention is to evaluate an educational programme or activity against existing standards, or to do research to discover new original knowledge. Evaluation focuses on a local programme, to assess how well the programme works. Information gathered during evaluation aids in decisions about modifying a programme to improve it. Research, however, aims to collect and analyse information in a way that will also transfer to other programmes in different places (Priest, 2001). If the intention is to describe or measure outcomes after the initiation of a new programme, an evaluation plan is needed. If what is required is an exploration of a new idea, or identification of themes about how service users and carers interact with learners in an educational setting, a descriptive research design is needed. If the intention is to test a specific intervention against a predetermined set of outcomes, an explanatory research design is required, such as a quasi-experimental or experimental design (Table 4.2).

Although many people tend to associate quasi-experimental and experimental designs with quantitative research and descriptive designs with surveys and qualitative research, this distinction does not always apply. Both descriptive research and experimental research can include either qualitative data or quantitative data or both. Once a question is determined, the domain of impact should be chosen. This will direct the outcomes that are to be observed, described, measured or tested. Once these are agreed, a design can be chosen. Many books provide detailed information about designing educational research and evaluation (Guba and Lincoln, 1989; Isaac and Michael, 1995; Kern *et al.*, 1998). The following provides brief summaries of designs.

4.5.1   Audits and Process Evaluation

Properly conceived, an audit and process evaluation can provide a good place to begin. This approach to evaluation enables those who plan and implement a new or modified educational programme to discover whether they have accomplished what they set out to do. A good process evaluation includes a clear plan with identified objectives that specify the programme components to implement and a timeline for implementation. The evaluators then document whether each step of the project and each component of the programme occurs, recording details about what happened at each step and whether the activity met the projected timeline. An audit may use checkmarks, tallies, verbal descriptions or numbers to describe what happened in each part of the project. For example, the Comensus project included a process evaluation. The participants reported whether planned activities occurred when they developed service user, carer and community involvement in health and social care education. They specified the activities that occurred during each phase of the project, identified questions that would enable them to determine whether the activities occurred as planned, and specified tools for collecting data to ascertain whether each component occurred and how it proceeded (Downe *et al.*, 2007).

4.5.2   Outcomes-Orientated Programme Evaluation

A programme evaluation that describes or measures outcomes provides systematic information about the effectiveness or impact of a teaching intervention or programme, informing decisions about whether to continue the programme or modify it in some way to better address objectives or meet programme goals. Even a thorough, systematic evaluation that addresses all the criteria for scholarship may not provide information that generalises to other programmes, as its

Table 4.2 Research and evaluation designs for education.

Designs	Purposes	Advantages	Challenges
Programme evaluation 1. Audits and process evaluation	To determine if a programme implemented components according to plan.	Documents what happened. Facilitates replication of a programme.	Requires attention to detail. Requires prospective planning.

2. Outcomes evaluation
  a. Participants' reactions
  b. Impact on learning
  c. Impact on behaviour
  d. Impact on organizations
  e. Impact on communities
	To determine (measure and/or describe) outcomes in a particular educational programme or setting.	Can determine whether a programme or a change in approach to education makes a difference. May help justify or obtain funding. Helps a programme modify what to do to achieve particular aims.	May be hard to define meaningful outcomes in a way that can be assessed.

Descriptive research (qualitative and quantitative) 1. Observations 2. Questionnaires and surveys	To describe characteristics, themes, patterns and relationships between aspects of a programme in a way that may generalise or transfer to other educational programmes or settings.	Builds understanding about approaches to education that can inform educational programme planning.	Requires prospective planning, including ethics committee review and approval. Requires a systematic approach. Requires expertise in research methods.

Explanatory research (qualitative and quantitative)
1. Theory generation and testing
2. Hypothesis testing
  a. Quasi-experiments
  b. Experiments
	To generate and/or test a theory, test an educational intervention, measure or describe change over time, and/or test cause and effect in a way that may generalise or transfer to other educational programmes or settings.	Builds understanding about the relationships between particular approaches to education and identified outcomes.	Requires prospective planning, including ethics committee review and approval. Requires a systematic approach. Requires expertise in research methods.

purpose is to evaluate a programme in a particular context. Hanson and Randall (2007a, 2007b) have described a simple approach to an evaluation in which the outcomes were the successful establishment of teaching activities that involve service users and carers in a medical school (in their terminology, 'patient and family advisors'). They assembled a large group of patient and family advisors, developed an innovative approach to co-creating new educational activities and described the activities that they successfully integrated in the teaching programme of the medical school. While these educational activities represented clear outcomes of the project, and they provided enough information that other medical education programmes could choose to implement the activities or a modified version of them, there was no attempt to develop generalizable information in the way that word is usually applied to research.

4.5.3 Descriptive Research

In descriptive research, educators use methods such as direct observations, questionnaires and surveys to describe characteristics, themes, patterns and relationships between aspects of a programme in a way that may generalise or transfer to other educational programmes or settings. Descriptive research helps educators uncover new insights, discover possible relationships, describe a point in time or change over time, describe experience, describe outcomes, generate questions or generate theory. Some categorise descriptive research as 'pre-experimental designs' (Campbell and Stanley, 1963). However, descriptive research can serve very useful and important purposes, particularly if the researchers give some thought to systematic generation of theory or questions for further study, and if evaluators push beyond descriptions of the process to descriptions of meaningful outcomes of educational work. Descriptive research designs include case studies without comparison groups, in which an educational programme or activity is described in detail, and one-group pre-test–post-test designs, where the investigators measure or describe participants' knowledge, skills, attitudes or behaviours before an educational activity, implement the activity with the group of learners who completed the pre-test, and then measure or describe the participants' knowledge, skills, attitudes or behaviours with a post-test or post-intervention set of observations. Another example of descriptive research is quantitative research that uses statistical tests of the correlations between different variables that have been measured in an educational programme. Correlations do not explain cause and effect, but they do identify relationships between the different variables.

Qualitative approaches to research may provide particularly useful tools for enquiry in educational programmes that engage service users and carers as teachers and curriculum planners. Qualitative approaches to research provide systematic ways to build understanding of the perspectives of people whose experience of life may be different from those of the investigator. 'Qualitative description' as a general research tool is useful (Neergaard et al., 2009). There are, however, several different approaches to qualitative research, each of which provides a set of tools to plan a study within a particular frame of reference. For example, constructivist research helps an investigator understand the ways people interpret social experiences, and how their social constructs shape their experience of life (Blumer, 1969; Magoon, 1977). In education that involves service users and carers, a constructivist approach would help a researcher explore how interpretations of social experiences shape reactions to and use of care and services. Ethnographic research helps build an understanding of cultures – such as the culture of people who need care for chronic health conditions, or the culture of people who seek care at a particular clinic or hospital (Schensul and LeCompte, 1999). Phenomenology seeks to understand a particular phenomenon from the perspective of one or more individuals. Phenomenological research is particularly useful when seeking to build an understanding of the meaning of an experience from the perspective of a particular group of people (Beaton and Clark, 2009). Grounded theory provides a way to approach data collection and interpretation that helps the researcher explain how themes that describe an educational programme or activity relate to each other, and to interpret and compare the data until a theory emerges from the researchers' interaction with the data (Glaser and Strauss, 1967). Helpful, comprehensive texts for qualitative research include those of Corbin and Strauss (2008) and Lincoln and Guba (1985).

4.5.4 Explanatory Research

Several designs are available to test a theory, test an educational intervention, or test cause and effect in a way that may generalise or transfer to other educational programmes or settings. In broad outline, designs may develop explanations by testing a theory, testing predictions, or testing the effectiveness of an educational intervention. No one study can provide completely definitive information that generalises to all settings but over time, when many studies contribute information about similar topics, a clear picture begins to emerge.

A researcher might test a theory devised from qualitative data by gathering additional qualitative data, looking for themes and relationships in the new data and then comparing the new data to the themes and relationships in the theory. If the data from new interviews, focus groups or observations support the themes and relationships described in the original data, this provides support for the theory. Over time, a theory can be modified to better represent qualitative data gathered in different settings or at different times. A well-developed theory could, for example explain how learning occurs in a medical education programme that includes service users and carers as teachers. A theory can also be tested with quantitative data. A researcher might, for example, form a theory about which behaviours or opinions fit in certain categories and then test the theory by gathering quantitative survey data and using statistical tests to identify sets of items that group together. A researcher could also test a theory by using a quantitative observation tool in different educational settings, to determine if observations in the different settings support a larger theory.

Another approach to explanatory research involves making predictions, usually considered a quantitative approach and tested with statistics. For example, a study could define and measure students' learning outcomes, and then test which aspects of service user and carer involvement in teaching best predict those outcomes.

The most familiar approach to explanatory research is to test a hypothesis using an experimental design. In this design, a study randomly assigns some participants to a group that experiences the intervention variable, which might be service users and carers sharing their experiences in healthcare with the learners. The experiment would assign approximately the same number of participants to a control group that experiences a traditional educational programme, with no service users or carers involved. For a true experiment, there must be prospective, completely random assignment to the two groups, and everything except the intervention variable should be the same in what the two groups experience. The study then measures the same learning outcomes for both groups and compares the results.

True randomization is usually not possible in educational settings, and providing exactly the same educational programme in every way except the one intervention variable is usually not possible either. For this reason, a variety of quasi-experimental designs have been developed. Campbell and Stanley thoroughly described many quasi-experimental designs in their classic book; Kern and Thomas have applied these designs to the development of medical education curricula and testing the educational interventions in the curricula. All of these designs have 'threats to validity' that the researcher must take into account but, when a researcher uses the designs carefully, they can result in useful information (Campbell and Stanley, 1963; Kern *et al.*, 1998; Colliver and McGaghie, 2008).

4.5.5   Systematic Reviews, Meta-Synthesis and Meta-Analysis

The literature includes several narrative reviews that address health professional education that involves service users and carers (Repper and Breeze, 2007; Wykurz and Kelly, 2002; Jha *et al.*, 2009a). Typically, there are not enough high-quality, quantitative studies in this literature, with similar statistical analyses, to enable a researcher to sum results across a collection of studies (Colliver, Kucera and Verhust, 2008). Neither are there enough qualitative research studies in the literature to enable someone to do a formal meta-synthesis of the findings of qualitative research regarding service user and carer involvement in health professional education. As more high-quality studies are done, our understanding will grow.

4.6   Research and Evaluation Methods

This section provides a menu of methods that are available to implement a research or evaluation design. In addition to thinking about which of these methods of data collection would best answer a particular question or outcome, it is important to consider what could be done most comfortably within a particular programme, institution and community context. Available resources, such as money or people with certain expertise, also play a role in the choice of methods.

Qualitative data collection gathers words and images. Retrospective data collection gathers existing documents or recordings, whereas prospective data collection follows a plan developed for a particular study and gathers new data. Options for qualitative data collection include the following:

Observation: Researchers watch people in the setting where the education they want to study happens. When planning the study, decide who and what to observe, where and when to observe, what to look for and how to record the data.

Interviews: Researchers ask questions of selected individuals, using open-ended and clarifying questions. When planning the study, decide who to interview, where and when to interview them, what questions to ask and how to record the data.

Focus Groups: Researchers ask open-ended and probing questions in groups of four to ten people. Again, plan who to include in the focus groups, where and when to hold the groups, what questions to ask and how to record the data.

Document Analysis: Researchers study reports, archived records, minutes of meetings, diaries and other documents and files. When planning the study, decide which documents to review, how to get access to them, what questions to ask when reviewing the documents and how to record information to analyse.

One classic text that explains how to apply qualitative methods to studies in educational settings is *Qualitative Research and Case Study Applications in Education* (Merriam, 1998). Inui and Frankel (1991) have articulated a helpful perspective for applying qualitative research in healthcare settings. Siwe and colleagues' (2006) qualitative study of women's experience of teaching the pelvic exam to medical students illustrates one of the key advantages of qualitative research – it provides a window into the perspective of a group of people with a shared experience. Building an understanding of any of the participants in a health professional education programme is a useful application of qualitative methods, as illustrated by this study. Researchers have used document analysis less often in educational work than interviews, focus groups and observations, but Cottingham *et al.* (2008) and Downe *et al.* (2007) provide two examples of incorporating minutes from meetings in qualitative studies of educational innovations.

4.6.1   Appreciative Enquiry

The concept of appreciative enquiry was initially articulated by David Cooperrider and colleagues in the 1980s as an approach to changing organizations through participatory action research (Cooperrider and Srivastva, 1987). They describe appreciative enquiry as an orientation to organizational change that is based on the fundamental belief in the human capacity for collaboration and creativity.

Rather than focusing on problem solving to repair deficits and failures, the appreciative enquiry approach involves the systematic discovery of what gives 'life' to an organization when it is at its best, and aligns those strengths to foster collaborative social innovation. The 'Four-D model' (discover, dream, design, deliver) is widely used to implement this approach. Participants work through the process of discovery of strengths by sharing stories of positive experiences; they build upon their discoveries by envisioning what might be, enter into dialogue about what should be and innovate for the collaboratively constructed future (Cooperrider *et al.*, 2000).

Appreciative enquiry has been used by groups of primary care physicians and patients with chronic conditions to discover 'best communication practices' in shared decision making to inform curricula (Lown, Sasson and Hinrichs, 2008; Lown, Hanson and Clark, 2009). Others have used an appreciative enquiry approach to foster culture change within an academic health centre (Cottingham *et al.*, 2008).

4.6.2   Participatory Action Research

Participatory action research provides a framework that emphasises participation of different stakeholders in the research (Wadsworth, 1998; Mills, 2000) and can be associated with empowerment or emancipation ideals (Carr and Kemmis, 1986). Critical or emancipatory approaches can be traced back to the liberationist influence of Paolo Freire (1971) (Chapter 2). Rather than thinking about researchers as distanced, objective observers of people or other objects of study, people engaged in participatory action research stay conscious of the active involvement of everyone engaged in and around a study. The Comensus project again provides an example (Downe *et al.*, 2007). In addition to 'active participation', people engaged in participatory action research think of research as a process of repeated cycles, rather than a linear process in which one step follows another in sequential fashion from the beginning to the end of the project. Each activity in the research process affects the other activities, from formulating a question to gathering some data, re-thinking the question, framing methods, gathering more data, revising hunches, interpreting, reaching tentative conclusions, asking more questions and so on, throughout the process of enquiry.

4.6.3   Observation Checklists and Rating Instruments

Like other methods, researchers can use observation checklists to collect quantitative or qualitative data or both, either checking off items they observe, writing comments and descriptions or rating items on a scale. In contrast to more open-ended qualitative research, however, observation checklists and rating instruments focus observations very specifically, so they are most useful when educators already know or have discovered the most important behaviours to observe or assess. Service users are involved in several well-established programmes designed to teach and evaluate clinical skills, such as communication and physical examination skills. In many of these programmes, they use observation checklists to evaluate specific skills. For example, service users with arthritis teach and evaluate physical examination skills using observation checklists in arthritis educator programmes. These programmes provide a good way to assess whether students have acquired behaviours that they can use as healthcare providers, as well as knowledge, after an educational activity (Raj *et al.* 2006).

4.6.4 Surveys and Questionnaires

A questionnaire is a written or computer-based tool that asks participants to answer specific questions. The requested answers can be either quantitative, such as ranking items in order or rating items on a scale, or qualitative, or both. Questions can be open-ended or focused. If a study uses a questionnaire to explore a topic, the researchers or evaluators can write questions tailored to their own interests and programme. In order to use sophisticated statistics and draw definitive conclusions, however, a study must use an instrument that someone has written and tested to see if the scores on the questionnaire really measure what they intend to measure, and do so reliably for the purposes of the study. The results of a survey will generalise to other settings if the instrument has been tested for reliability and validity, and one samples participants in a systematic way that accurately represents the study target group. Many resources describe how to develop and use questionnaires and surveys (Fink and Kosecoff, 1985; Woodward, 1988; Rea and Parker, 1997).

4.6.5 Emergent Methods

Educational programmes and activities require creative approaches to research and evaluation. Studying the impact of programmes on attitudes, behaviour, performance outcomes, cultures and communities requires innovative ways of viewing evaluation. While traditional experimental research that controls and manipulates variables helps build an understanding of which educational interventions result in certain outcomes, natural teaching environments make it difficult to isolate and control variables. Often educational work is better served by qualitative research, appreciative enquiry and participatory action research, all of which provide ways to conduct a study in the context in which education occurs. Even these research approaches as they have been applied in other studies sometimes do not provide the range of methods needed to conduct an enquiry about a new educational approach, so researchers may find themselves in need of innovative approaches to research. It may be necessary to combine research methods in a creative way or consider new methods that have been used less often, such as those described as 'emergent methods' (Hesse-Biber and Leavy, 2008). For example, Lown and colleagues (2009) combined appreciative enquiry, qualitative research methods and teaching strategies in pairs and workgroups to gather the data for their study of shared decision making, involving both physicians and patients in each teaching/learning/data collection session.

4.7 Data Analysis and Interpretation

When planning for data analysis and interpretation, thinking about practical details early in the project will simplify the process later. For example, consider the following: What data will the study generate? What system can the project put in place to ensure that future replication of data collection and analysis will be possible? Who will take responsibility for collecting, managing and analysing the data? Will the study require qualitative or quantitative analysis software, audio or video recorders, tapes or other supplies? What team members will you need to observe, assist, interview, transcribe, distribute questionnaires or analyse data? Will you need an expert in qualitative analysis or statistics, and who will that be? What, specifically, will you do to analyse the data, and who do you need on the analysis team?

Many comprehensive textbooks are available to describe the details of data analysis; the ones noted here are just samples that cover a variety of approaches: Corbin and Strauss (2008) describe qualitative data analysis; Tukey (1977) details exploratory data analysis with quantitative data; and Newton and Rudestam (1999) offer an easily-understood introduction to statistical data analysis.

When interpreting the results of data analysis, it is especially important to ensure that people with a variety of perspectives participate to enhance understanding of the results in relation to the purposes and goals of an educational programme. When the team thinks back to the purposes of the project and the questions they posed at the beginning, its members will decide together not only what the results mean, but also who needs to hear about them, how to present them and what next steps in education and evaluation will help everyone move forward together.

4.8 Planning and Implementing Research and Evaluation

Appendix 1 provides a planning worksheet to guide decisions about a research or evaluation project, from choosing domains of outcomes and writing questions, to choosing a research or evaluation design, selecting methods for data collection, analysing and interpreting data, and sharing findings with others. While the worksheet includes all the components one would plan in a research or evaluation project, it does not represent a process in which a researcher would start at the top of the first page and work through it in a precise order. Most research and evaluation projects will change and take shape over time. Careful planning becomes even better when the members of the team learn from each other and gather insights as the study proceeds, adjusting the research and evaluation process as the process unfolds. This is part of 'reflective critique', which is one of the essential components of systematic scholarship. Thoughtful educators reflect at the beginning of the project when planning what domains to assess and how to construct a project, and throughout the project, learning from the research and evaluation process as well as from the results of the study.

4.9 Conclusions

Programme evaluation and educational research about service user and carer involvement in health professional education presents both challenges and rewards. Participants' experiences and perspectives are not easily described, and the many variables that affect teaching and learning in complex social systems make such work complex. Nevertheless, we encourage all who value service user and carer involvement in health professional education to assess their work using the menu of designs and methods described in this chapter, and to select those most appropriate to each context. Clarify your vision, articulate the gap between what is and what might be, plan and implement educational programmes to address the gap, assess the impact, reflect on results and share them so we can build on each others' work. By sharing our insights, we can begin to co-create theories and models for learning, and to study the impact of service user and carer involvement on attitudinal, behavioural and social change in healthcare. By doing so, we will build an international community of educators and learners committed to including the perspectives, experiences and expertise of service user and carers in health professional education.

Definitions

1. *Patient teacher* – a person who teaches students in the health professions, teaching from his or her perspective as someone who has been a recipient of healthcare.
2. *Patient advisor* – a person who advises in regard to development of teaching activities, curriculum design, research agenda and design, evaluation strategies, and/or interpretation of evaluation or research data, speaking from the perspective of his or her experience with healthcare as a patient.
3. *Parent teacher* – a person who applies his or her experience with healthcare to teaching students in the health professions.
4. *Parent advisor* – the parent of a child with special healthcare needs who advises in regard to development of teaching activities, curriculum design, research agenda and design, evaluation strategies, and/or interpretation of evaluation or research data, speaking from the perspective of his or her experience with healthcare as a parent.

5. *Research* – systematic investigation that aims to add to generalizable or transferable knowledge or understanding.
6. *Evaluation* – systematic development of questions and collection of data designed to ascertain the effect or usefulness of a programme or intervention.
7. *Scholarship* – systematic study that aims to discover new knowledge, teach and develop new approaches to teaching, apply knowledge to socially important issues or integrate knowledge across disciplines. Scholarship involves asking questions, setting goals, designing an enquiry or project, evaluating, critiquing, submitting the work to peer review, and disseminating findings.

5 What Counts Cannot be Counted: Community Engagement as a Catalyst for Emotional Intelligence

> Each of us occupies each other's position at some stage in the past, or the future, and we are interested in making this as good as it can possibly be.

5.1 Introduction

Previous chapters in this book have described the social and theoretical context for service user and carer engagement, and methods and techniques for evaluating success. The levels for programme evaluation proposed by Kirkpatrick (1998), described in Chapter 4, offer a useful taxonomy for categorizing outcomes into satisfaction with the programme itself, knowledge and skills learned, behaviour change or skill development and tangible outcomes as a consequence of the programme. Although Chapter 4 gives examples of projects that can be logged against each of these levels, a recent review in this area (Morgan and Jones, 2009) has noted that most studies of community involvement in higher education have concentrated on process measures, which are not a part of Kirkpatrick's taxonomy, or outcomes relating to immediate gains by the service users or students (satisfaction scales, and personal development/knowledge transfer). Longer-term outcomes, including changes in skills and behaviours, and improvements in tangible outcomes for future service users, are not often reported in evaluations of engagement projects. At the very least, this critique demands an examination of the theories and philosophies underlying professional education, and the fit between these factors, and the results of engagement activities.

In this chapter, we describe potential stakeholders in service user and carer engagement in higher education. We examine the kinds of outcomes that might matter to these groups. Then, in recognition that the outcomes debate needs to be reframed by theory, we use Benner's novice to expert model (Benner, 1984) and Kohlbergs moral reasoning taxonomy (Kohlberg, 1973) to try to understand the purpose of higher education for the health and social services. We arrive at the conclusion that there are two clear axes in the health and social care professions, one focused on practice, and one on attitudes and values. Using two paradigmatic accounts of engagement, we suggest that service user input is a crucial element of the attitude and values axis, and that outcomes attributed to this engagement should be focused in this area.

Based on the work of Hills and Mullett (2000), we debate the tension between an ethical stance that sees engagement as a moral good in itself (standing outside the need for formal outcomes-based justification) and the knowledge–economy imperatives of universities in a world where reaching targets and standards is the prime driver. We then turn to a description of the general move in health and social care from researcher-defined outcomes based on theories of ill health, to those that are defined by service users themselves. We specifically examine interpretations of health and well-being that move beyond pathologising disability and social disadvantage. Using the UK Medical Research Council (MRC) model for the evaluation of complex interventions as a starting point (MRC, 2008), we return to an examination of the theoretical basis for engagement and, as a consequence, the nature of the unique contribution of engagement for universities.

We accept that a part of the purpose of engagement strategies is simple awareness raising about a range of specific health and social care conditions and circumstances. However, we move beyond this, to consider the issue of emotional intelligence. Based on the accounts given throughout this book, and in other relevant papers, we propose that the strong narrative element of engagement is a powerful catalyst for the transmission of complex salutogenic ideas. Measures of emotional intelligence in students and staff exposed to this input might provide a framework to compare the effect of different approaches to engagement, but only if these are not reduced to linear numeric scores. We examine new methods of assessment that take account of the complex, emergent, salutogenic nature of engagement outcomes, and that account for the unique perspective of individuals, as well as for the need for standard comparisons at the population and organisational levels.

5.2   Defining the Stakeholders

The constituencies for service user and carer engagement in higher education are usually characterised as those who take part in engagement activity, and the students and teaching staff they have direct contact with. There is less material relating to the wider community from which service users and carers may be drawn, to institutional concerns, to commissioners of education and of health and social care services, or to the impact of engagement projects on future users of health and social care services. In the latter case, this is more because of the difficulties of attribution of service user and carer input during training to specific clinical outputs down track.

The omission of the wider community, and of organisational and commissioning stakeholders, is more puzzling. There can be a taken-for-granted view that universities stand apart from the communities in which they are situated, as reflected in the commonly used phrases 'town versus gown' and 'ivory tower'. Despite the reality being more complex than this, such tensions have been highlighted in scoping work undertaken at the beginning of at least one engagement project that has been comprehensively examined in this volume (Downe *et al.*, 2007). The imagined or real hostility engendered by this split has potential adverse consequences, both in terms of accessibility to higher education for local communities, and in terms of knowledge transfer, commercialisation of ideas, and dissemination of cutting edge innovation from higher education institutions (HEIs) to local businesses and services. Partnerships between universities and local communities are encouraged in the United Kingdom by the governmental Widening Participation agenda and the Economic and Social Research Council (ESRC) research programme on the impact of universities on regional economies (ESRC, 2009). This funds the formation of partnerships between universities and community groups to benefit student education and experience through community-based research and user forums.

Community engagement also needs to be understood in terms of mutual learning between universities and communities. There is clear support from some funders to provide a more holistic and critical interpretation of the impact on local communities which will enable the benefits to be demonstrated (ESRC, 2009). This does not preclude the need for critical appraisal of community engagement projects. There is a risk in assuming that engagement is inevitably a positive activity. However, active engagement with community groups without a history of university attendance might be one way of building bridges and opening up opportunities into and out of universities. This stakeholder group is, therefore, vital for effective service user and carer engagement.

Private businesses and institutions are highly and directly motivated by the opinions of their core users, as this is the best way of maximising profit. The marketisation of public commissioners and institutions, and, specifically, the rhetoric of consumer choice, have forced an increasing responsiveness in public organisations, at least at a superficial level. The modernist target-led culture that is a feature in many countries has necessitated an organisational focus on issues handed down as important drivers by governments. Governments change every few years in most jurisdictions, so this focus can be transitory, but sometimes all parties agree with an issue and it gains more longevity. Service user and carer involvement seems to be one of these factors, at least in some countries. As a result, health and social care personnel commissioning agencies have become major stakeholders in the service user and carer agenda. This, in turn, has led to at least nominal attention from universities, which must deliver on the targets of the commissioning bodies.

While the political move towards engagement as a norm and not an exception is to be welcomed, the risk is a tick box response, where one or, at the most, two individuals are invited to a few meetings and left to cope (or not) on their own. The more subtle effect might be that genuinely authentic engagement initiatives, which entail active support and training and are almost inevitably more expensive, are suppressed on the basis that enough has been done and no more is needed. Simple process outcomes may indicate that tick box engagement has been successful. However, this is unlikely to fulfil the aspirations of all the other stakeholders in this enterprise, and is very unlikely to have long-term effects on health and social care well-being. In the next section, a consideration of the theoretical underpinning for outcome measurement in this field is discussed.

5.3   What Outcomes Matter?

There appears to be little agreement on the outcomes that matter to a range of stakeholders, and which can effectively assess the impact of service user, carer and community engagement. The few standard outcomes that have been proposed do not appear to be based on theoretical constructs or formal evidence of their reliability, validity, responsiveness and of when they should be assessed. The impact of service user engagement at all levels of Kirkpatrick's taxonomy (Kirkpatrick, 1998) may resonate for many years after the initial encounter with students, or input to a validation board, or contribution to a research project. Most formal process and personal development evaluations of new innovations in this area, as in most others, are funded in the early stages of an innovation, and not at the later stages, when a more mature model may have evolved, with better processes and outcomes.

In one of the few studies that have attempted to identify the outcomes that matter to service users and carers, Barnes, Carpenter and Bailey (2000) focused on assessing 'added value' by developing a questionnaire comprising user-developed outcome indicators, which was verified by a second user group. This study of interprofessional learning concluded that the outcomes that service users prioritised included:

- Students should demonstrate understanding, not just try to solve problems or push people into services.
- Students should treat service users with respect, not as labels.
- First and foremost, professionals should develop their capacity to 'be human'.
- Students should have knowledge about services, including advocacy services and service user groups.
- Students should be able to provide information about how to involve service users in assessing their needs.

Another study by Masters *et al.* (2002), which focused upon the evaluation of a project from strategic level to implementation, investigated the perspective of all stakeholders. The service users in this study felt that they benefited from learning new skills, from increased self-confidence and from a genuine feeling of empowerment. In all of the above studies, service users valued being active participants in developing the humanistic skills of students, and in experiencing increased 'power sharing'. It appears that there is a strong desire from service users and carers who engage with health and social care education to improve services for themselves and for future recipients by helping students understand and care for people at a personal, human level (Turner *et al.*, 2000). This, in turn, allows service users and carers to be seen as individuals in all aspects of their lives, whilst breaking down stereotypes of passivity and enabling damaged confidence to be rebuilt (Costello and Horne, 2001).

From the perspective of the university, outcomes are focused on: student satisfaction and academic achievement (and consequent future student recruitment and retention); quality control of timetables, course approvals and modes of assessment; and fulfilment of the targets set by funders and governments. In some cases, local, national and international reputation is also important, especially if this increases income from research and development sources. The potential conflict between these imperatives and the outcomes seen to be important by service users might generate a tension between the 'ideal' of user involvement taught and the 'grim reality of practice' (Masters *et al.*, 2002). Even where these outcomes are apparently in alignment, such as the UK governmental demand for service user input into social work education, they may conflict at the operational level. Having nominal input that meets audit standards is not a guarantee that the outcomes desired by service users themselves are achieved.

There appears to be little evidence about the outcomes that would be valued by educational staff or students who are the recipients of service user and carer input. Research undertaken within specific projects indicates that students generally find the participation of service users and carers a positive experience (Turner *et al.*, 2000; Costello and Horne, 2001). It appears to enhance the learning experience, as students gain a greater understanding and empathy leading to informative and instructive teaching sessions (Turner *et al.*, 2000). Wood and Wilson-Barnett (1999) conclude that the early involvement of service users and carers in teaching programmes may be more effective in terms of influencing teaching. In most cases, students appear to value the opportunity to gain real life experiences instead of hypothetical cases, although a minority can feel embarrassed and inhibited by the presence of service users and carers (Costello and Horne, 2001). However, the outcome measures used in these studies do not appear to be systematically derived from the student perspective. This is an under-researched area that requires more examination in future.

There is even less reported on outcomes that might measure the longer-term impact of university service user and carer engagement for the future recipients of care. Historically, outcomes in medical research have tended to be based on a positivist paradigm that values minimisation of bias and simplification of interventions. In the early medical publications, participants were referred to as 'materials' and then as 'subjects'. This linguistic turn expresses the relationship between those doing the research and the researched. Although research methods in the social sciences have always been more reflexive, the outcomes of health and social care have, until recently, been largely researcher determined, with little or no attention paid to the experiences of service users and carers. There is an increasing interest in so called 'patient-led' outcomes, but these still tend to be based on a limited set of variables which, in turn, are conceptually restricted. Many are focused on the relief of pathology, rather than on the generation of well-being; for example, the SF36 (SF36.org, 2009) and the Hospital Anxiety and Depression scale (Zigmond and Snaith, 1983). Even those based on individual experience tend to be standardised, with 'satisfaction' measures being a prime example. As Haas (1999) has noted, the concept is underdeveloped. Indeed, surveys of user satisfaction appear to consistently record that around 80% of people are satisfied, even though a significant minority of these individuals will report poor quality care and dissatisfaction if they are then offered the chance to discuss their experiences in in-depth interviews.

Over the last ten years or so, the term 'participants' has replaced 'subjects' in research reports, and alternative and more nuanced evaluation tools have been suggested to capture some of the subtleties of the experiences of users and carers. Quality of Life (QoL) measures are a classic example of this new genre (Higginson and Carr, 2001). These methods of assessment are based on a list of factors that are deemed to matter to service users, such as activities of daily living. Sometimes the list is researcher derived, and sometimes it is generated by qualitative work with a group deemed to be representative of the population being assessed. However, there has been criticism of the reductionist nature of these tools, as the list of items in the scale may not be relevant to certain individuals, and the final outcome is a statistically derived single numeric score, often translated into a proxy economic measure, like quality adjusted life years (Qualys) (Pliskin, Shepard and Weinstein, 1980).

The publication of the Patient Generated Index (Ruta, Garratt and Russell, 1999) offers a conceptually revolutionary approach to generating Quality of Life scores. The tool asks respondents to list anything at all that matters to them in relation to the topic being assessed, and then derives population level Quality of Life scores from the listed items. This means that each person taking part has a uniquely individual basis for the final score that is derived. In the last decade a series of studies of an adapted version of this tool for maternity services (termed the Mother Generated Index) has demonstrated its validity and reliability (Symon and Dobb, 2008). There is no reason why this approach cannot be adapted for all the stakeholders in the service user and carer engagement arena.

At the same time as reductionist population-based outcome measures have been under scrutiny, there has been a growing critique of the negative phrasing of many clinical outcome measures. The positive psychology movement is an example of the resistance to the classically pathological framing of mental illness, for example. It has been noted that service users and carers often do not perceive of their circumstances negatively, and they resist labels such as 'vulnerable' or 'fragile' (Downe *et al.*, 2009). Indeed, many in these circumstances overcome extreme pressures and setbacks every day. Many are not merely overcoming ill health and poor social conditions, but they are achieving positive well-being. In 1948, the World Health Oganization (WHO) said that *'Health is a complete state of physical, mental and social well-being and not merely the absence of disease or infirmity'*.

The work of Hills and Mullett (2000) offers an unusually theoretical take on community-based research that provides a nuanced basis for well-being as a core output of community engagement. The authors argue that community-based research is fundamentally participatory, that it encompasses an ontological reciprocity between the self and the social and physical environment, and that it prioritises practical, presentational, empirical and experiential knowing. From the point of view of Hills and Mullett, this generates a unique theoretical basis for community involvement that is fundamentally concerned with praxis, as a 'reflective relationship in which both action and reflection build on one another' (Hills and Mullett, 2000: p6). They go on to argue that, axiomatically, the value of this kind of approach is human flourishing: *what is of interest is more than the usual research outcome. The utility of the outcome is judged based on what difference it makes to transforming the health and wellbeing of the community'.*

Returning to the definition of stakeholders, the community that benefits from engagement may encompass a wide range of players. The range of outcome measures to be used in this context should ideally capture this eudemonic (happiness-based) turn. Concepts of salutogenesis (Antonovsky, 1987) and of resilience (Barnes and Morris, 2007) are able to do this; this is returned to later in this chapter.

5.4   The Purpose of Health and Social Care Education

There does not appear to have been any comprehensive theoretical analysis of the fundamental components of effective health and social care. Scrutiny of the Internet sites of the organisations responsible for validating educational programmes in the United Kingdom, such as the Nursing and Midwifery Council, the General Medical Council and the General Social Care Council, reveals lists of competencies or skill sets. It is a similar story for the composite benchmarking statements articulated by the UK universities' Quality Assurance Agency. International sites, such as the International Councils of Nursing and of Midwifery, or the International Federation of Obstetricians and Gynaecologists, give either statements that encompass a general scope of clinical work or sets of standards around attitudes and behaviour. A bipartite clinical/attitudinal model seems to be prevalent in professional accounts of health and social care practice. In most cases, the attitude/values aspects are listed before the clinical/skills ones, suggesting that the former are of primary importance. Recently, Cohen has claimed that, in a medical context:

> Professionalism denotes a way of behaving in accordance with certain normative values, whereas humanism denotes an intrinsic set of deep-seated convictions about one's obligations toward others. Viewed in this way, humanism is seen as the passion that animates professionalism. (Cohen, 2007: 1029)

Indeed, there is growing evidence that empathic attitudes in healthcare providers can affect service users' immune system functioning and hasten recovery from illness (Rakel *et al.*, 2009).

The assumption seems to be that validated programmes are effective in transmitting both the clinical and the attitudinal/values aspects of this ideal scope of practice to students. There does not appear to be any systematic method of assessing this across health and social care groups. In the apparent absence of a consistent and coherent theoretical basis for health and social care education, general learning theory might be an appropriate source of guidance. This tends to fall into the realms of behaviourism (what people do, what can be observed), cognitivism (how people think) and constructivism (development of novel modes of thinking and of seeing and understanding the world). For behaviourists, learning is the acquisition of new behaviour through conditioning. Conditioning can be expressed in a Pavlovian sense (the programming of an automatic response based on repeated exposure to the same experience) or on 'operant' conditioning, noted by Skinner (1957) and based on reinforcement or punishment.

Health and social care education that is based on passive learning styles and on assessment by grade alone tends to be orientated towards behaviourist theories of learning, and to the notion that professional education is primarily about acquiring knowledge and skill sets.

Cognitive theories of education are based on the gestalt psychologists, who emerged in the late 1920s (Bode, 1929). This approach sees learning as being based on pattern recognition and whole pictures of events, as opposed to the rote learning of decontextualised facts and behaviours. Identifying patterns of events and consequences leads to the capacity to extend understanding to new situations that have not been encountered before. The work in this area includes examination of learning how to learn and social role acquisition. Problem Based Learning (PBL) has a basis in cognitive theory (Savin-Baden, 2000; Chur-Hanson and Koopowitz, 2004). It has been used to develop subtle and sophisticated skills in solving complex clinical and social care problems, but is less often overtly designed to foster empathy, humanism and compassion.

Constructivist approaches move beyond cognitive pattern making, and into the capacity to create new and unique knowledge and understanding, based on interactions between the individual and their social and physical environment. Educational techniques based on this theoretical construct can lead to profound (and sometimes, for the individual, disturbing) shifts in values and beliefs. New approaches to professional education, such as narrative-based learning (Greenhalgh and Collard, 2003), reflective practice (Schon, 1983) and transformational learning techniques (Cranton, 1994), depend on constructivist ideologies. It is in this domain that attitudes and behaviours might most effectively be challenged and changed.

5.5   Addressing the Attitudinal/Values Axis

It appears, then, that the professional project of most health and social care professions is founded both on practical knowledge and skills, and on the expression of humanistic and altruistic attitudes and values. In one of the few comprehensive models of professional development in the field of healthcare, Benner (1984) has adapted the novice to expertise model proposed by Dreyfus and Dreyfus (1986) for the nursing context. The model is not profession specific. The original authors derived their theory from a study of chess players and airline pilots. As a framework for health and social care, the basic taxonomy can be applied across the health and social care disciplines. It proposes a move through five stages, from Novice, through Advanced Beginner, Competent, Proficient and, finally, Expert.

In terms of the theories of education explored above, the movement can also be characterised as a shift from a more behavourist approach, where the novice is responsive to rules and formal performance standards, to a more cognitive stage of competence that can move beyond fixed rules to a choice of action from a range of possibilities. In the later stages of the model, the individual can progress to a greater degree of emotional involvement, and an apparently intuitive response that is constructed in action by the particular environment and social/professional situation in which experts find themselves. Practitioners in the later stages of the model are reflexive (Schon, 1983) and more likely than those in the earlier stages to take creative risks based on the particular situation as it presents itself. Their actions appear to be intuitive, but they are, in fact, dynamically drawing from previous experience and from a vast store of knowledge and skills.

The material from which expert general medical practitioners build their diagnoses has been termed 'illness scripts' (Eraut, 1994). These scripts can be constructed solely from previous clinical encounters. However, they are more likely to include other elements alongside clinical experience, including stored knowledge and contextual details, such as the impact of the social circumstances of the presenting service user. This is mediated by the service user/doctor relationship that may or may not have been developed in past encounters. It is likely that the scripting process operates in many professional encounters. It is possible that one of the unique features of health and social care scripts might be the development of a moral sophistication that in turn informs the attitudinal/behavioural axis of professional practice.

Kohlberg's (1973) theory of moral reasoning provides a useful analysis of the move from simple (level one) to complex moral awareness (level 6) (Box 5.1).

As in the model of Dreyfus and Dreyfus (1986), Kohlberg argues that individuals move sequentially along this continuum, becoming increasingly able to apply judgement to moral situations. There are criticisms of Kohlberg's theory, mainly focused on the exclusive focus on judgement as an arbiter of moral reasoning. However, as a heuristic, it provides a useful basis from which to understand the development of the attitudinal aspects of health and social care education.

5.6   Developing the Moral Practitioner: Story as Praxis

Given the general lack of a theoretical explanation for health and social care practice, we return to the practice/attitudinal domains as the best focus for educational

Box 5.1   Kohlbergs Levels of Moral Reasoning

	View of Persons	Social Perspective
6	Persons are ends in themselves and must be treated as such.	Moral point of view: mutual respect as a universal principle.
5	Recognise that contracts will allow persons to increase welfare of both.	Contractual perspective: considers moral and legal point of view; recognises they sometimes conflict and finds it difficult to integrate them. Resolved by formal agreements.
4	Able to see abstract normative systems.	Social systems perspective: differentiates between societal point of view and interpersonal agreement or motives.
3	Recognise good and bad intentions.	Social relationships perspective: Aware of shared interpersonal relationships, feelings and expectations, which take primacy over individual interests. Putting yourself in other person's shoes.
2	Sees that (a) others have goals and preferences, (b) either conforms to or deviates from norms.	Instrumental egoism: Serves one's own needs but is aware of others' interests and conflicting interests.
1	No view of persons: only self & and norm are recognised.	Blind egoism: does not consider the interests of others or recognise that they might be different from one's own.

Adapted from Kohlberg (1984: 174–176). Reproduced with permission of Elsevier.

effort in this area. The range of skills and knowledge-based criteria and assessments described in textbooks, and embedded in curricula, implies that the practice aspects of professional education are well developed. In contrast, apart from formal sessions on communication, and on theoretical ethical principles, many professional programmes, and most health and social care textbooks, give little formal space for the development of a moral and ethical sensibility. The need for morally responsible values and empathic behaviours may be taken for granted as a good in themselves. This creates the risk that these aspects of health and social are assumed to be inherent, and that education systems do not need to engage with them. This may risk the production of health and social care practitioners who are technically competent, but ethically and emotionally deficient.

As noted above, there is increasing evidence that empathy, as an attribute based on a moral sense of the need to see the humanity in others and to do the best for them, might have measurable physiological consequences. For example Nummenmaa *et al.* (2008) have recently demonstrated that emotional empathy has profound neuro-physiological consequences for the person feeling empathic. This orientates them towards *somatic, sensory and motor representation of other peoples' mental states*

(Nummenmaa *et al.*, 2008: 571). Emergent findings like these give further impetus to the search for methods to expose and challenge the moral, ethical and emotional responses of health and social care students and practitioners.

Service user and carer engagement might be a primary route to the development of the values and attitudinal axis of professional practice. In the experiment above, empathy was stimulated by the use of photographs. Two examples of teaching and learning included in this book illustrate how empathy is generated through service user engagement (see pages 151–154). In the first example, experienced staff were exposed to assessment of their capacity to deal with practice situations that might demand restraint of service users, by a service user who had herself been restrained. The initial wariness of the students implies that they were aware that exposure to scrutiny from outside of the comfort zone of professional peers might force them to rethink their normative approaches. In the end, the experience was overwhelmingly positive, and possibly even transformative, for both the professionals and the service user involved. For some in this group, who had been practising for some time, the disturbance caused by dissonance between their normative practice and the insights arising from the service user narrative might have been enough to re-set their moral compass. This is an example of moral development based on a constructionist educational approach.

In the second account, two letters tell the chronological story of a service user who has a history of self-harm and alcohol misuse. In this case, the audience is undergraduate students who are learning to set their moral and empathic compass in the context of clinical practice. It provides an example of a theoretically grounded approach, based on narrative, designed to produce reasoning based on the complex emergent phenomena of an individual life, and not on linear reductionist analysis.

5.7   Towards a Unifying Theory of the Effect of Service User Engagement

Service user engagement is a complex intervention, on the basis of the Medical Research Council (MRC, 2008) definition that a complex intervention is one with several interacting components. The Medical Research Council proposes that evaluation of complex interventions should not be based on single, clinically defined outcome measures, but on an understanding of the theoretical constructs that underpin these interventions, and then on modelling of the impact of the overall package before the final detailed evaluation is carried out. Just as it is important to locate a theoretical basis for professional practice and education, there is a need to identify such a basis for service user engagement. The question arises as to whether engagement is a moral good in itself, or if it must be subject to the knowledge–economy imperatives of universities in a world where reaching targets and standards is the prime driver.

We have argued that the theoretical basis for engagement is the potential to fill the moral and ethical gap in current provision, focused on the of attitudes/values axis of health and social care provision. In order to maximise this potential, we would theorise a need to move from seeing service users and carers as vulnerable or fragile, and in need of paternalistic professional support. Insights into the resilience of people and families who can create positive families and communities under the extreme pressures of illness, disability and deprivation offer the potential to see service users as guides and mentors, and not as dependent sufferers (Werner and Smith, 1982). Service users and carers who tell stories of tragedy and triumph illustrate the salutogenic focus described by Antonovsky (1993):

> A salutogenic orientation facilities seeing things that experts in a given pathology might well fail to see ... it ... pressures one to think in systems terms ... it leads one to deal with (both) entropic (disorder-promoting) forces and ... negentropic (order-promoting) forces.

Outcome measures that assess the impact of salutogenic stories on longer-term delivery of healthcare need, in themselves, to be salutogenic. Rather than measuring degrees of suffering and pathology, measures of increased well-being and self-esteem are more likely to capture the effect of authentic engagement, where it is embedded in, and normative for, a university. These measures also need to capture the interconnected and emergent nature of engagement as a dynamic process that has multiple internal feedback loops. As engagement is seen to work, positive feedback spreads to the student body and the educational staff, generating more interest, more engagement and more positive effects. This process is illustrated in Chapter 6. As problems and issues are faced and overcome, so the system develops self-knowledge and an increased capacity to overcome problems in the future. The increased positive outcomes again feed back to generate the will to increase engagement in the future. The engagement process is, therefore, a complex adaptive system. Such systems tend to be dynamic creative and attractive (Plsek and Greenhalgh, 2001).

Ultimately, it seems that one of the primary results of service user engagement might be to increase emotional intelligence (EI) in all the stakeholders who take part. For the purpose of our argument, we combine the definitions of Salovey and Mayer (1990), who understand EI to be a combination of emotional perception, emotion use, understanding of emotion and emotion management, with that of Bar-On (2006), who defines EI as being concerned with effectively understanding oneself and others, relating well to people and adapting to, and coping with, the immediate surroundings, in order to be more successful in dealing with environmental demands. There is a considerable debate and critique around the nature and measurement of EI, some of which is academic sophistry, and some of which expresses a genuine concern that the field of EI might be falling into a reductionist trap. However, the kind of behaviours that appear to be present in those who are highly emotionally intelligent are also those that were identified by service users in the study by Barnes, Carpenter and Bailey (2000) discussed above, and in the higher levels of the moral reasoning taxonomy of Kohlberg (1973).

We propose that the strong narrative element of engagement is a powerful catalyst for the transmission of complex salutogenic ideas, and that measures of EI in students and staff exposed to this input might provide a framework to compare the effect of different approaches to engagement. Techniques for measuring this outcome in students and staff that are based on the individual/population approach of the Patient Generated Index (PGI) (Ruta, Garratt and Russell, 1999) might solve the apparently irreconcilable dichotomy between standardised measures that fulfil the external assessment of universities and person-specific aspects of self-development. These kinds of measures could also be used to measure increased resilience and salutogensis in the lives of service users and carers who take part in engagement activities. Using the PGI itself to assess longer-term outcomes for those cared for by students who have experienced engagement will allow for the identification of the specific health, social care, personal and well-being factors that matter to each individual service user, and for QoL comparisons across cohorts. All of these theories and techniques could provide a coherent model of evaluation for the future. Using subtle models of data collection to assess the development and impact of EI, based on complexity, salutogenesis and the unique point of view of individuals, might, finally, allow us to count what, before, could not be counted, and, in counting it, express its value coherently. This may be a powerful vehicle through which universities can transmit the missing attitude/values axis of professional practice.

> Not every patient can be saved, but his illness may be eased by the way the doctor responds to him – and in responding to him the doctor may save himself. But first he must become a student again; he has to dissect the cadaver of his professional persona...It may be necessary to give up some of his authority in exchange for his humanity, but as the old family doctors knew, this is not a bad bargain. In learning to talk to his patients, the doctor may talk himself back into loving his work...by letting the sick man into his heart...they can share, as few others can, the wonder, terror, and exaltation of being on the edge of being, between the natural and the supernatural. (Broyard, 1992)

Part II: Personal Experiences: The Case of Comensus

6 Setting up a Service User and Carer Engagement Project: Comensus

It was very nice when I initially started with Comensus. I was told that I would only have to go at a pace that I was comfortable with. I have been coming to meetings and other diverse learning and teaching opportunities which have made my brain work... [it is] like throwing a pebble into a calm pond and it just seems to grow.

6.1 Introduction

This chapter focuses on the practicalities of developing a service user and carer project within higher education. Comensus is a whole-Faculty approach to service user and carer engagement. The chapter is written from the perspective of the Comensus project coordinator. It illustrates the practical day-to-day events and lessons that arise from putting the rhetoric of engagement into practice. The tables and appendices provide tools and processes that might be of interest to other individuals and groups with such projects planned or in progress. In Chapter 7, the lessons from complementary processes, developed in a single School, nursing, are examined. Both chapters illustrate routes taken to try to ensure authentic, systematic and integrated service user and carer involvement in higher education. The emergent nature of such engagement processes can be deduced from the accounts given in these two chapters. While both projects were subject to careful planning at the outset, the final route taken was not always the one that had been predicted. This was often as a consequence of the organisational culture in which Comensus was situated.

The project is based within a university in the North West of England, in the Faculty of Health. The Faculty educates future and current health professionals, including nurses, paramedics, midwives, doctors and social workers. As noted in Chapters 1 and 2 of this book, United Kingdom health and social care services all have a remit to put patients at the centre of care, and require services and practice to be person centred. Government legislation also champions user involvement and patient-centred care (DH, 1998b, 2000a, 2000b, 2001a, 2005, 2006a, 2007). It has extended this drive to include the commissioning of health and social care education.

The university set up the project with this one aim, of systematically involving users and carers in all scholarly activity within the Faculty. This is done in a variety of ways, with service users and carers contributing to the development of teaching materials, being involved in teaching and assessment, being involved in research and having a presence on the many committees that contribute to the work of the Faculty. The project is in itself a vehicle for cultural change within the Faculty. Although it can be seen as a discrete entity, it is still subject to, and influenced by, the academic world in which it is based. It has an institutional identification and is susceptible to the forces that impact on the larger institution. The notion of culture is particularly pertinent to Comensus as its work, like all similar initiatives, has to strive for a place in an already established culture that has long established norms and rules.

> Significant modernization in user participation is occurring requiring momentous cultural changes that are intended to transform the traditional inert role of users to one of autonomy and active participation. (Bradshaw, 2008: 674)

6.2   Background to Comensus

Before Comensus started there was a degree of service user and carer involvement within the Faculty, but piecemeal and uncoordinated. Early attempts to improve this state of affairs included the establishment of a Faculty interdisciplinary group of academics interested in issues of user involvement. This group had representation from nursing, midwifery, social work, post-graduate medicine and the Centre for Ethnicity and Health; the latter developing a reputation for supporting community engagement processes (Fountain, Patel and Buffin, 2007). It was energy that developed within this grouping that led to the university investing the necessary resources to establish Comensus.

The project was initially commissioned in 2004 for three years. Comensus was initiated as a participatory action research project, so that future activities could be formed out of action cycles. The premise of action research is that the processes and output of the project evolve cyclically. Activity is planned – it takes place – the effectiveness of the processes and the utility of the result are reviewed – from the findings, the next stage is planned (Carr and Kemmis, 1986; Reason and Bradbury, 2000; Lewin, 1946). Choosing this approach ensured that the project developed according to the needs of its members and of the environment in which it was placed.

Unlike service user and carer engagement initiatives in other universities, Comensus had a full cohort of staff, including a project coordinator (full time), an administration assistant (18.5 hours per week), a research assistant (15 hours per week) and two experienced academic researchers (who gave their time according to the needs of the project). The coordinator and administration assistant were tasked with the practicalities of day-to-day activity, and the research assistant was tasked with supporting research and reporting to the team. The more experienced academic researchers had split roles, one being responsible for supervision of the research assistant, and the other having responsibility for support and development of the project and its staff members. Both academic researchers were responsible for project-related research activity (such as supporting the writing of papers and presentation of findings at conferences).

6.3   Beginnings

The staff team all had an ideological commitment to authentic service user and carer involvement. They did not want to appoint service user/carer representatives to the project without help, guidance and advice from local community representatives, support from university staff already carrying out community engagement activities, and help from statutory service staff who were committed to the success of a service user and carer initiative that would engage with future practitioners. It was for this reason that the creation of a community Advisory Group was planned from the outset, with the intention of making the project authentic and meaningful. To enable this to happen the project coordinator spent time visiting community groups to allay people's fears, answer people's questions and raise awareness about the remit, value and ethos of the work proposed. Individuals who showed an interest in the work, and those who were resistant, based on previous negative experiences with the university, were invited to the first meeting of the group at which terms of reference were discussed and agreed, and the Advisory Group was officially set up. The terms of reference for the group are given in Appendix 2.

The Advisory Group members were made up of representatives from local voluntary sector organisations, statutory services and academics from the Faculty of Health. All members had experience of service user and carer involvement and were committed to the development of an authentic meaningful project. Members offered expertise, acted as a sounding board and ensured good practice was developed from the start. The power within the project at this time resided with the Advisory Group, as it made the major decisions and directed project development. The Advisory Group acted as a team and the outline of the project started to develop. In the spirit of developing reciprocal relationships between the university and community groups, all non-statutory groups with personnel attending advisory group meetings received on honorarium of £50 per meeting.

The Advisory Group and staff team officially launched the project in April 2004 by holding a pre-recruitment open day for service users and carers. The day was used to elicit responses to three specific areas. These topics were discussed by participants within workshops. All participants were informed of the intention to set up a service user and carer group for the project (later to be termed the Community Involvement Team, or CIT).

Those attending workshop one were asked the question, in which aspects of the Faculty of Health's work should service users and carers be involved? The responses were that they should: help to plan, check and provide teaching and training in the university and the community; be involved in all parts of research to make sure that the work belongs as much to service users as to university researchers; and the group members should take part in course and Faculty development by being part of making choices and linking with communities.

Workshop two focused on how the group should be set up and run. The consensus was that membership should be open to anyone who has used health and social care services. Relevant participants should be found by going out to groups and/or by organising a bigger event in the future. To permit the development of skills and knowledge, people should be on the group for one or two years. Group members should be responsible for reaching out from their own groups, making sure that everybody uses everyday language, and signing-up to a mission statement. The group should meet every two months at first, then every three months. At these meetings people should share the work, so that only one task is done by one person. They should also work as a focus group. The group would need to meet in community settings and at the right time for members. They would also need clerical support, training, respite care for carer members, information in everyday language, buddies and support from Faculty of Health staff at all levels.

Workshop three focused on ways of finding out how the group (and the wider Comensus project) was working. It was agreed that key outcomes should be that the project/social firm existed as a good, well-known and copied model. People would feel that they were supported, equal partners, whose skills and job chances were better for taking part. There would be better health and social care services, planned and provided by people who were more suitably educated. Everyday language would be used by all. The project would not just be about the issues of one or two specific user groups.

Those attending the workshop felt that the methods of assessing this success needed to be valid and reliable. They agreed that people should be asked what they thought, and service users should be asked if services are better. The number of people who have been trained and employed because of the project, and the amount of service-user input should also be counted. Knowledge of the project, use of the group by the Faculty and taking-on of ideas by other Faculties should also be measured. The people to ask if Comensus was working should include service users and Comensus service user and carer group members, students and teachers, Comensus workers (including the Advisory Group), people in the community and service providers (statutory and voluntary).

Wider issues also came out of the workshops on the launch day. These included:

- The university does not have a good reputation locally. 'Townies and students' are two separate entities.
- The university consumes land and buildings.
- When people have engaged in the past they have not been recognised within reports and papers for their input.
- Information should be accessible. This included a call for the use of everyday language, not jargon, in all outputs of the project.

- The university and the community should work together as partners and equals, as *'Engagement brings together different types of expertise'*.
- More information from research and user group activities undertaken at the university should be shared with the community.

In its first year, the Advisory Group considered and debated a number of the matters arising from the workshops. The issues and activities of the project at this stage in its development are described in Downe *et al.* (2007). Appendix 3 details these key issues with corresponding decisions and solutions.

Over a ten-month period, the Advisory Group worked through these issues, finding the solutions set out in the second column of Appendix 3. At this point, the Advisory Group was ready to recruit service users and carer representatives. An open meeting was held in February 2005 to answer any questions those considering applying for a place on the CIT may have. From this event, 24 applications were received for group membership.

6.4   Research Activities

As previously discussed, Comensus staff included academics with a research remit. The task at this juncture was to map service user and carer involvement across the Faculty. The Faculty staff was interviewed in relation to this mapping exercise. It reported a lack of awareness of the range of service user related activities that were taking place across the Faculty (and, indeed, a lack of knowledge of the Comensus Project itself). This exercise found duplication of effort, and the development of some isolated initiatives that were tapping into the same local voluntary and community sector resources. This was deemed to have a negative influence on perceptions of the university (as evidenced in verbal reports/comments to Comensus project staff). Comensus responded to this situation by hosting an information sharing/group working away-day for all key service user 'active' staff.

It was whilst driving home from this event that the first Comensus coordinator, Eileen Johnson, had a road accident and tragically died. As can be imagined there was some disruption to the course of the project and colleagues felt that a respectful pause was in order before advertising for a new coordinator. The present incumbent eventually took up the post roughly six months from Eileen's passing.

6.5   Development of the Community Involvement Team

The Advisory Group put application forms together, appointed an interview panel of service users and carers, and began the process of recruitment. It successfully recruited 21 individuals from diverse backgrounds. Members' expertise and personal experience included physical disabilities, mental ill health, HIV/Aids, drug/alcohol misuse, learning disabilities, experiences of being carers for children with complex needs and carers of the elderly. Members also belonged to different cultures and different faith groups.

The first meeting was held on 8 March 2005. Three key issues emerged from the discussion, mirroring some of the issues identified in the service user and carer literature, as discussed elsewhere in this book.

Representation emerged as an important issue, mirroring the debates in this area amongst professional staff. The group members debated who they represented. Did they only offer personal opinions, or should they stand for others in their position? The group decided at this stage that members were just representing their own views. This was, in fact, the original expectation when the project was initiated.

It is agreed widely (Turner and Beresford, 2005; Involve, 2006) that service users and carers should be reimbursed for expenses and, where possible, paid for the contribution of their time and effort. However, these payments are dependent on a number of factors. These include internal systems that allow for flexibility of payment, the funding of the initiative and the participant themselves and their ability to accept payment. (Payment may not be allowed for those claiming certain welfare benefits.)

Good practice indicates that users should be paid where possible in cash on the day of involvement. Payment should be discrete, saving embarrassment for participants all of whom should be guided to seek welfare benefit advice. Reasons for payment include the recognition and the value afforded the participants in the involvement opportunity. Payment also addresses equity issues, power relationships and directly impacts some key barriers to participation, such as carer costs or travel expenses.

Within Comensus the debate over payment has been fraught. One dilemma faced was that whilst all concerned recognised that there should be equity of payment with other academic partners, the resources within the project were not sufficient to enable this to be carried out if authentic and widespread involvement was called for. When the Community Involvement Team was first set up this was a significant focus for discussion amongst the members. The members decided democratically that their preference would be for involvement to be systematically paid at the maximum rate the project could afford whilst maintaining authenticity. Along with this, however, members themselves reflected on their reasons for involvement and decided their main motivation was not payment but the chance to make a difference and get their voices heard in a way that is not tokenistic. Comensus strives to pay equitably and in some cases (especially where outside funding is identified) this does happen, usually following the university rate for ad hoc lecturing fees; however, this is not the norm. This issue is still being debated and, whilst this method works for the CIT at the time of writing, this may not always be the preferred option and it is revisited frequently. All out-of-pocket expenses are covered, and an additional monthly amount of non-receipted expenses is available for CIT members to reflect the myriad ways in which expenses can be occurred in the ongoing work of the group. Interestingly, not all members opt to receive these sums; some prefer to be seen as providing their input on a voluntary basis. Others donate payments and/or expenses to community groups to which they are affiliated; and these transfers are made directly. All payment issues, including the necessity to defray expenses on the day of involvement have caused headaches with standard administrative forms and payroll requirements. These issues have been largely resolved in dialogue with the relevant departments. The consequences of payment strategies for individuals were also discussed, specifically, how payment to take part in Comensus might affect benefit payments. It was agreed that a welfare rights agency should be contacted locally to give advice. Group members were encouraged to check out their position, and a series of welfare rights surgeries have been held on campus for group members.

The explicit provision of emotional support was seen to be a vital ingredient for the successful operation of the group. It was noted that some members might require extra support, and ways of providing this were discussed.

Other support needs identified by those present included not using jargon, establishing ground rules and ensuring comprehensive minutes were produced. The group also spent some time identifying its training needs, and discussing how research interviews could be carried out with (rather than on) members. Terms of reference of the group were agreed over the next few meetings (Appendix 4).

The second meeting of the group focused on the processes of the project, dealing with administrative decisions and looking at how people wanted to be included. As the group was so diverse, there was the potential for divisions at this stage. Some members commented that 'the pace is frustrating but necessary', but others felt definitively that 'the work is too slow'. The newly appointed coordinator was an expert in community work, but had no prior experience of working in an academic environment. In the light of the frustrations expressed at the progress made, the first task of the new coordinator was to review activity so far, to work with and get to know the members, and to understand the culture of the organisation. This was not always straightforward:

> It was like making eggs on the moon, I was familiar with the processes and understood clearly the tasks involved but carrying this out in the Faculty where the majority of people were unfamiliar with service user/carer involvement meant I was constantly defending my right and the right of the project to be there. (Lisa, Comensus Coordinator 2005)

Felton and Stickley (2004) note that, *'the notion of service users as teachers challenges perceptions of the role of 'mental health lecturers' as the experts'*. They go on to discuss the nature of power in education, seeing it as a key element of the culture of pedagogy. This would suggest that the maintenance of this power is important for teachers whether they acknowledge it or not. These norms were implicitly challenged by the Comensus project, in general, and the coordinator, in particular.

In an attempt to overcome these fears, the coordinator spent a large amount of time visiting Department Heads and identifying academic champions who could help to promote service user and carer involvement across the Faculty. To promote engagement from the education staff, a 'Celebration Event' was also held. This promoted the benefits of service user and carer involvement for teaching staff, and raised awareness of the processes involved.

As recommended by Wykurz and Kelly (2002), the coordinator and the Community Involvement Team members devised a package of support that could be put in place for those members taking part in teaching opportunities. The CIT members who were planning a teaching session would spend time with the coordinator discussing the teaching opportunity in detail. This included an examination of the remit and nature of the involvement opportunity and the make up of the student cohort. In each case, a meeting was arranged with the academic who requested the involvement, so that the CIT members could acquaint themselves with the subject and plan accordingly. The Community Involvement Team member would be given the opportunity to visit the classroom before the session so any accessibility requirements not already discussed could be met. The coordinator was always available on the day of the session, and for emotional and practical support after the event, to ensure that emotional distress did not occur as a consequence of the involvement opportunity.

This level of support was offered to all members regardless of experience, as the CIT decided that they all were susceptible to bad days, and would rather refuse help on the day should they wish to than not have the help offered at all. Training on presentation skills was commissioned for CIT members from a service user-led training group (GEM, Giving Experience Meaning). In a general sense, all participants invested time and energy into developing relationships within the group, raising the possibilities of peer support and establishment of friendships rather than just working relationships (Chapter 2). On top of this, the CIT's activities always included time for social events, which were important for bonding and stress relief.

Unfortunately, at this stage involvement opportunities were sparse, with the main involvement requests coming from the Mental Health Division of the Department of Nursing. This Division was the first to accept Comensus as integral to its work. It invited the project to be part of its strategic decision making processes through having an equal voice on the divisional team, invitations to validation meetings, recruitment involvement and inclusion as equal partners on many module teams. Some of the members with other conditions and different experiences felt that the project was not delivering the possible opportunities that were available within the Faculty. The coordinator raised this within Department (now School) Executive Team Meetings, Divisional Team Meetings and one-to-one meetings with academics. Progress was slow, but eventually inroads were made into academia.

A pivotal event was the Quality Assurance Agency (QAA) major review of nursing programmes. Comensus had been invited to meet with the reviewers, who were impressed with the project and could see its potential. The good review of the project's contribution was celebrated within the Faculty and new involvement opportunities began to be requested. Another major factor in the success in developing the project was the work of the community and academic champions, who raised awareness and opened up opportunities for the work.

The Faculty began to see the value of the project and started to engage the CIT more comprehensively. This included invitations to attend Faculty Disability

Advisory Groups, Faculty Executive Team meetings, open days and recruitment events, Student Experience Committees, Department and Divisional Meetings, Faculty Ethics Committee, Academic Standards meetings, and the School of Nursing Service User and Carer Forum.

Although engagement was now happening, it was not organised or strategic. At this stage, the CIT came together and devised an action plan for the coming year (an example of action planning is given in Appendix 5). It was agreed that the plan would be reviewed and built upon through coming years until the CIT could confidently say that involvement in the faculty was systematic and integrated.

6.6   Rhetoric or Involvement – CIT One Year In

At the end of the first year of the operation of the CIT, logistical barriers within the faculty had been overcome, and a system of expense payment had been devised so people could be paid to get to and from meetings without it affecting their benefits. Funding was also available if people had additional support costs associated with attending meetings, or needed to pay for a carer at home so they could be free to attend. Information was being produced in a wide variety of formats, and a full package of training was set up to support the CIT in its endeavours. Venues for CIT meetings were shared around between university rooms and various community settings.

Despite the fact that the CIT was getting increasingly more involved in activity, it still faced many challenges at this stage. Although internal meetings within the project were accessible and jargon free, this was not always the case during other meetings. The group felt more confident amongst itself and with its activities. However, it found it difficult to fundamentally change the format of other people's meetings and the academic and bureaucratic systems within the Faculty.

The scope of involvement was also different within the various Schools across the Faculty. Some of the Schools were well on the way to becoming partners whilst others were still wrestling with the notion of involving service users and carers in teaching. The CIT decided to carry out a major marketing campaign to promote service user and carer involvement. It designed posters, leaflets and a Web site (www.uclan.ac.uk/comensus) and developed a good practice guide for service user and carer involvement. This handbook outlined how to engage and support service users and carers. The group took this work one step further and designed an Accessible Writing Guide, which provided suggestions for academics and students on how to write documents and presentations using accessible language and pictures. All of this work provided exemplars of good practice, but did not have the desired effect of substantially increasing engagement of the Faculty staff. It appeared that the barriers were too complex to be immediately overcome with these kinds of approaches.

By this point, the CIT had developed a strategy group whose remit was to examine the direction and scope of involvement, and to guide and progress the project.

This group decided that all activity should be evaluated, and tasked a working group to develop appropriate forms. It was felt that dissemination of the results of evaluation (if it was good) might create a positive feedback loop that could increase future engagement. The evaluation process included:

- Student evaluation forms – for students to give feedback on particular teaching sessions.
- Academic evaluation forms – for academics to give feedback on the process from initial enquiry with Comensus to engagement with students.
- Service user/carer evaluation forms – for individuals to report on their involvement. This form was used also to identify personal development and training opportunities and give feedback on practical and logistical issues.

The strategy group also looked at other quality assurance mechanisms and started to hold twice-yearly quality circles. These are informal individual or group meetings with staff to comment on the things people liked, things they didn't like, current activity and future developments. CIT members were also able to give feedback after all CIT meetings to the research assistant as part of the ongoing action research process. All feedback was discussed and acted upon and contributed to the action plan for the forthcoming year.

6.7   Comensus – Year 3

In the third year, activity started increasing across all disciplines within the Faculty. CIT members were constantly engaged in teaching, and other opportunities for involvement were increasing. As confidence built in the CIT, work began on developing and writing a CIT module on service user and carer engagement for a Foundation Degree in Health and Social Care. Other new activities included developing problem based learning packages, developing new DVDs covering mental health issues and learning disabilities to be used in teaching, developing interactive learning materials for interprofessional learning and writing case scenarios for the social work department.

At this stage, the CIT were becoming thinly spread across the wide range of activities being developed. They recognised the need to revisit the idea of sub-groups as a useful division of labour, these being smaller groups that could focus on specific work streams. Earlier incarnations of sub-groups had been useful in the initial development of the CIT's work, but had somewhat lapsed as the core CIT meetings had become more efficient. Appendix 6 describes these sub-groups, and their remit.

Although all of these groups had a specific remit and devolved responsibility, all final decisions had to be fed back to the wider CIT for discussion and ratification. This model of working suited the ethos of the project. Members were all involved in decision making. They could do as much or as little as they liked; they had the chance to learn new skills; and they could focus on topics that interested and excited them.

The positive energy generated by all these activities was considerable. It was not all plain sailing and project staff were worried about the amount of work in which some people were engaged. Furthermore, this take-off in work levels coincided with the final year of project funding for Comensus. Indeed, on reflection, it seemed that CIT members were trying to carry out as much activity as possible in the time the project had left. The workload issue was examined and, in the event, it was clear that it was manageable. The staff team, the CIT, the Advisory Group, Faculty staff and management all realised that, because of the delays the project had faced and the potential value of the work, funding needed to continue. As a result of intense lobbying from all these groups, the project was commissioned for another year. The continuation of the project, however, was not decided with certainty until very late on in the year.

6.8   Issues and Solutions

This third year was pivotal for Comensus. The team faced a wide range of issues and new challenges. Solutions that would accommodate the members yet meet the requests from academics for involvement were identified in collaboration. Appendix 7 describes this process.

6.9   Comensus as a Social Firm

One of the initial aims of the Comensus project was to work towards establishing a social firm to be the vehicle for delivering service user and carer contributions within the university. It was anticipated that this would have to be on the basis of significant internal funding, matched with an equally substantial external grant, before self-sustaining contracting into the future could be considered. The initial ideas were developed together with the Advisory Group, but were quickly taken over by a sub-group of the CIT, with concentrated planning and exploratory work being undertaken in the third year of Comensus. It was intended that the development of the social firm would be conducted in a participatory, action context – comprising a development partnership between the university and service user groups and other interested stakeholders. There was no predetermined blueprint, rather it was wished to grow the project òrganically, and evaluate its success as part of the development process, utilising action research approaches.

Initially, some key features or goals of the development were anticipated:

- An organisation managed independently of the university.
- Constituted as a not-for-profit business – surplus income being ploughed back into the operational costs and development of the firm.

- Employing and being run by service users with one possibility being a cooperative structure.
- Developing model employment practices in the course of setting up the firm.
- Individuals being waged at levels on a par with other university employees.
- An important element being the provision of capacity building training for the social firm workforce; looking to develop accredited modules/certificates/diplomas.
- Exploring ways of assisting people to make the transition from reliance on statutory welfare benefits to waged employment.
- Using model working practices that balance the benefits of paid employment with the stresses of work.
- Supporting individuals prone to relapse of mental ill health, without losing them from the firm. This will require model sickness/absence policies.
- Aspiring to integrate the firm to wider community (state and voluntary sector) schemes for advancing individuals into employment or further education and training.
- Innovating links to other opportunities for mainstream employment – so individuals who have developed their capacity within the firm can exit to other jobs or education opportunities, for example becoming an employee of the university or local health/social care provider.
- Linking to widen access (and provision of appropriate support) to enable individuals to participate in the range of university courses – including professional training for health and social care disciplines.
- Capitalising on flux in the firm's workforce to avoid reifying the notion of 'service user', allowing people to develop mainstream employment identities.
- Establishing links with trade unions: for example supporting individuals who have lost previous employment due to health problems; working with peer groups of workers to ensure individuals are fully supported when making transition back into work.

Local support and development agencies linked to the Advisory Group helped the ideas to be developed. This involved a degree of facilitation and information gathering with a large sub-group within the CIT. It was the intention from the outset that the whole process would be fully participatory and any emergent social firm would be effectively owned and governed by service users and carers themselves. Despite much collective effort to develop these ideas, undertake market research and write grant applications, a number of factors conspired to defeat the aspirations to build this sort of social firm. Firstly, many of the eventual participants in Comensus could see both advantages and disadvantages in securing full independence from the university. As such, the 'risk' attendant on a more business-like model was unappealing. Others were, and still are, quite taken with the confidence and esteem that came along with working in the university, and liked the idea that they belonged to it in some way. Perhaps, along with this was the inevitable building of friendships and relationships with university personnel, and close involvement in meetings and such like that militated against considering a greater degree of independence. A bigger and more obvious obstacle was the strong sense of altruism and voluntarism evident in the behaviour of many, perhaps the majority, of participants who simply did not want to undertake paid work in a formal and organised sense. Ultimately, however, it has been the failure to secure a decent size grant which has been the major impediment, together with some possibly fatal flaws in the envisaged business model.

Any nascent social firm would have to persuade other groups and institutions to buy its services, with the major contractor being the university itself. The market research showed that other external groups were keen on the sort of resource that could be provided, but much less interested in, or able to, consider paying for it at the level needed to sustain the business. Similarly, the university, in times of financial constraint, has been reluctant to consider shifting its approach to paying for this form of participation. One area of resistance is a belief that paying people through Comensus as a Socal Firm represents a duplication of funding, without significantly demonstrating the promotion of substantive user posts and employability. In effect, the university would have to increase its financial commitment to contract for a range of user and carer inputs. This increase in monies would make possible the realisation of the major social benefits, notably employment opportunities. Despite universities being relatively rich organisations within their communities, and however desirable, this leap might be a step too far, at least in the prevailing economic climate in the United Kingdom.

6.10   Year 4 – On the Road to Strategic Involvement

Core work was carried out within the project throughout year four. Teaching activities, strategic involvement and development of a range of new learning materials in different media continued. The project had been promoted widely. However, activity was still not integrated equally across all of the different disciplinary teams within the Faculty. To rectify this, the CIT and the project staff examined activity across the faculty and identified gaps. As part of the action planning for the year, the team decided to concentrate on the gaps and to raise the skills of staff within the Faculty to support service users and carers they consistently work with. This would leave Comensus staff free to concentrate on new activity. Activity for Comensus 2007 focused on two other major areas; firstly, to identify future funding and, secondly, to develop and host a service user and carer involvement conference focusing on higher education. This had the title *Authenticity to Action*, recognising the increasing concern in the project that both authenticity and action were pivotal to the success of initiatives like Comensus.

6.10.1   Funding and Resources

Comensus funding was still not assured beyond the next year, and staff had been tasked with identifying outside funding opportunities. The staff and the CIT felt that funding applications should only be made for grants and funding that complemented the core work of the project, or contributed to the development of that work. A small grant tendered by Skills for Care North West was successfully secured. The application was for the development of seven two-hour lesson plans focusing on a number of key topics arising in social work education. The unique approach offered by the Comensus bid was that the topics would be delivered from a service user and carer perspective, to ensure that authentic voices would be heard in the teaching and learning process.

The seven teaching sessions and associated learning materials were prepared to address the following important issues in social care:

- User and carer involvement in social care policy and critique.
- Equality, diversity and user and carer involvement.
- User and carer involvement in assessment of need.
- User and carer involvement in delivery of social care.
- User and carer involvement in a context of risk management.
- Participation as a social movement: transforming social care.
- Staff and user alliances: how to maximise user and carer participation in the workplace.

Development of the lesson plans was a time consuming and challenging process. Before embarking on writing up the topic content, discussion took place across the team of CIT members and Comensus project workers about the ethos and values that should be imparted. The difficulty was that the text had to be written such that the product could be potentially delivered by other higher education establishments, so it was important that the underlying philosophy was clear in the materials produced. Given that the intention was to provide an explicit user/carer perspective on the issues, some people felt very strongly that the work should not shy away from some of the contentious material in subjects such as risk assessment.

In the event, the group was very innovative in the teaching methods adopted. The final teaching pack used a combination of audio, case study and visual media. The lesson plans were piloted in late 2008 to over 100 University of Central Lancashire (UCLan) Social Work Masters Students. Feedback was very complimentary, with comments such as *'enhanced my knowledge and will make a difference to my practice'* (MA Social Work Student, 2008) common across the lessons.

Comensus was also successful in obtaining grant funding in partnership with Bradford University to build a virtual online community. The Bradton[1] e-learning resource is a virtual 'town' populated by people who have used health and social care services because of various health conditions and/or related social needs

---

[1] The Bradton project has been developed primarily with Learning, Teaching and Assessment funding from the University of Bradford and a Harris award for excellence in research informed teaching from UCLan. The virtual learning resource can be found at: http://bradton.pbworks.com

and/or assumed an informal caring role. Experiences are presented as DVD or audio clips backed up with transcripts by service users or by simulated patients. The main aim of the project was to promote a person centred approach in health care education through collaboration with service users and carers, by producing learning materials that students are able to access online. The intention is to enhance and not replace valuable 'face-to-face' contact between students and service users through the use of individual's stories in an online environment. Individual personal experiences are linked to specific learning scenarios which complement and support health and social care practitioner teaching for use across a variety of courses and modules.

Other grants have included 'Sandbox'[2] monies for enquiry into the potential for peer support between health and social care service users and carers to be enhanced by digital technologies. This project explored the need for peer support and communication with participants from two established community groups in Preston: mental health service users and informal carers. The project team provided creative facilitation of focus groups to explore how the project should be framed and used interactive demonstrations of technologies to find out what format each group would prefer to use for its communication/peer support needs. The project has identified a 'blueprint' for peer support and communication systems for each group. The findings suggest that participants are greatly enthused and see a number of benefits of utilising technology for these and other creative ends, not least in tackling key issues of social isolation. Some of these include interesting observations on personal value and identity. Participants are, however, concerned about such issues as privacy and security and recognise certain personal training needs and workload commitments to maintain an online effective system.

The other major activity in 2007 was staging the *Authenticity to Action* Conference. This was led by a steering group made up of academics from a range of universities in the United Kingdom and service users and carers. All of those in the team were involved in reviewing the abstracts, were responsible for decisions about bursary applications and were actively engaged in contributing to the overall design and development of the conference. Beresford and colleagues (2006) speak of how being treated as an equal can really change the culture of workers and organisations. This view resonated with Les Collier, one of the service users involved in the organisation of the conference:

> As a mental health service user I felt equal to other colleagues which in many places does not happen. I felt I could take an active part without fears of any sort.

In preparation for taking on these roles, training was provided, support was available and encouragement was given throughout the process. These projects

---

[2] Sandbox (http://sandbox.uclan.ac.uk) is a UCLan interdisciplinary facilitation space and R&D laboratory for enquiry into digital technologies. It has also been a source of seedcorn grants to foster relevant interdisciplinary research.

can be time consuming for support workers and all involved. However, the outcomes are always worth the effort, and the conference was really well received and attended, with around half the audience coming from a user or carer perspective.

6.11   Tensions in Comensus

Engaging in outside activity connected to Comensus is always invigorating. The team has been lucky enough to be engaged in some very interesting and groundbreaking work. However, this externally funded work does take the staff team and the CIT away from core activities in what is an already busy project. The necessity of this engagement is undeniable with resources at a premium. However, the possibility of over-burdening participants has to be taken into consideration. It is also important to reflect on the remit of the project, and whether additional work detracts from core aims and, potentially, causes a challenge to the values of the project.

6.12   Year 5 of Comensus Activity

Following the exertions of the conference, the CIT and the Comensus staff decided they needed to be more strategic in their future involvement. From this point on, activity was planned around the anticipated outcomes that would be delivered, against the project objectives. Action planning became more focused on strategy, and on identifying and meeting gaps, with core activity assuming a central concern. Communication and liaison with management and outside bodies was also highlighted, as was planning activity to ensure demand does not exceed resources. Core work carried on throughout the year with the CIT contributing to:

- Planning of courses including new BSc Nursing and Nursing Diploma courses.
- Contribution at a number of validation events.
- Development and delivery of a seminar on user and carer involvement.
- The production of a number of resources, including DVDs on mentorship and the role of the service user in the relationship and Interpersonal skills from a service user and carer perspective.
- The production of two DVD comic skits on service user and carer involvement in education to be used in promoting Comensus.
- The production of a short film looking at why people get involved in service user and carer involvement – 'What it means to me'.
- The production of a film festival focusing on mental health awareness and anti-stigma, using the University's own cinema and, hence, opening this up to the community.

Other major developments came from the members themselves who, over the years, had become more skilled and more confident. This led to a change of practice with increasing numbers of the group chairing meetings, taking and producing the minutes and running and planning the meetings. Practice between the members changed, with support coming from peers rather than the onus being on the project coordinator.

Comensus at this time was asked to support the activities of SUCAG (Service User and Carer Advisory Group), a social work focused service user and carer project attached to the BA and MA programmes within the social work division of the Faculty. This project evolved out of the General Social Care Council (GSCC) recommendations that service user and carer involvement should be present in all stages of the design and delivery of social work programmes. The GSCC identified core funding to support the work, and financial ring-fencing of these monies was one of the reasons for having a distinct user and carer involvement initiative within social work. This paid for staff time and for the payment of service users and carers, resourced the project adequately, allowing activity to focus on core work and removing the necessity to identify extra project funding and other income-generating external activities, enabled the project to develop and gave it the prospect of realistic continuity.

This new arena brought challenges and anxieties for both groups. Discussion was needed to address fears that each initiative would lose its specific identity, the need to accommodate to changes in involvement practices, and the best way of adapting to different approaches to support processes. The SUCAG group was also losing its development worker, who had been assigned to another project. It made sense for SUCAG to become a partner group of Comensus, as some activity was duplicated and there were already established relationships. SUCAG had its own brand and way of doing things. For example, payment of expenses was set at different rates from those pertaining in Comensus and the types of involvement activity were in some ways dissimilar. Both groups discussed this individually within meetings, and the consensus for both was that it would be a good idea to come together despite these differences. To date, this has been a successful collaboration.

6.13 Stability

As is clear from the chronology above, Comensus suffered as a consequence of being seen initially as a time-limited project. This led to annual crises in planning, both for the project workers (who did not know if they would have a job from one year to the next) and for the CIT members. Given the feelings of the local community when Comensus was being planned, that the university had previously acted in bad faith with respect to engagement projects, this uncertainty raised real fears that the project would be closed down just as it was beginning to make a significant difference. Each year, persistent lobbying ensured support for the next year.

Eventually, in 2008, Comensus was funded recurrently as part of the core activity of the Faculty. Even though there is a continuing requirement to seek external funds for at least part of the work, this assurance of permanency is a testament to the success of the project, the CIT and Advisory Group members, and the project workers.

6.14   Year 6 of Comensus Activity

Comensus activities in 2009 have included working in partnership with Rethink, the national mental health charity, to facilitate and support service user and carer involvement for the North West Mental Health Improvement Programme (MHIP). These activities concentrate on eliciting views on mental health services from mental health service users and carers from across the North West. The Group organised another *Authenticity to Action* conference in November 2009 and another Film Festival in October 2009.

A continued focus on core work has been complemented with new developments, particularly within the social work school, building on previous activity by SUCAG. Part of the process of Comensus and SUCAG becoming partners included evaluating activity and putting processes together for systematic involvement. This started with a focus on the Masters programme. A joint decision was made with service users and carers, the Head of School and the course leader to treat involvement in the MA as a pilot that could be rolled out to other courses, to ensure activity that is authentic and not tokenistic and also evidence capacity building. The process started by mapping current activity across the Masters programme, specifically looking for duplication and gaps. Then all possible service user and carer involvement opportunities were identified, along with optimal ways of generating engagement. The next step was to look at how strategic decisions are made and then to look at power and partnership working, and this work continues. It is at an early stage in the process and it is envisaged that it will take 12–24 months before it can actually be said that service users and carers are fully integrated in the course. This is a very important piece of work, as it has not been possible to carry out such an intensive plan before, focused on a discrete aspect of course provision. We are realistic in what we can achieve and recognise that we can change how we are involved and some of the processes, but integration does not necessarily mean a change in the culture. That is a bigger piece of work.

6.15   Back to Beginnings

Service user and carer involvement is complex. This chapter started by highlighting cultural issues that impact on the development of authentic engagement. This section returns to those issues, in the light of the events in Comensus that have been described above.

In the university that is home to Comensus, staff generally agree with its mission statement. The organisation has a strong identity and vision, and these are reinforced for staff from recruitment to retirement. This is seen by some as good practice.

In effect, the university has a strong culture. Strong cultures have entrenched assumptions, beliefs and values; they use specific language, they refer to organisational legend, and they objectify certain symbols. Individuals in strong cultures demonstrate behaviour and habits that fit the nature of the organisation. These behaviours are not accidental or happenstance.

Comensus has the assignment of incorporating new values into the existing culture. The group is tasked with involving service users and carers in all aspects of scholarly activity and with changing the power dynamic within the existing overarching culture. But the university is also hierarchical, bureaucratic and cumbersome in some of its processes. Although the Faculty leader has a belief in the ethos of service user and carer involvement in higher education, and the values of engagement are clearly expressed in the university's vision and rhetoric, the reality is that this value has not been authentically taken up by some staff.

Despite some subtle but powerful resistance evident over the first five years or so of the project, Comensus' members have recently noted small cultural shifts, in that the project is now being welcomed inside the strategic arena of the Faculty. New values are being espoused, and the status of the project and the commitment it receives from managers is slowly changing for the better as these values become absorbed into the existing cultural hierarchy. Aspects of relational culture have also been affected where service users and carers have begun to work closely with certain individual staff members or teams and communal and formal spaces are increasingly inhabited by Comensus members. It is in these relationships, possibly, that shifts in such identity issues as how people are seen, and how they see themselves, can change for both service users and staff alike.

The experience of Comensus is that it might not be necessary to enforce all five of Pennington's (2003) criteria to develop effective engagement (Chapter 1). The final two criteria, making change a way of life and creating opportunities for ownership, might be the most important catalysts for authentic cultural change in this regard.

7 Climbing the Ladder of Involvement: A Manager's Perspective

Nigel Harrison

We began by feeling our way along and now we are able to lead the way.

7.1 Introduction

This chapter offers a personal reflection on the process of service user and carer engagement from my perspective as Associate Head of a large School of Nursing and Caring Sciences. I am designated with lead responsibility for service user and carer involvement across curriculum within both the School and the Faculty of Health and Social Care. These responsibilities involved appreciable transactions of liaison and mutual support, between activity at the School level and the Faculty-wide contribution of the Comensus initiative.

While this is my own personal perspective, I recognise that my views have been influenced by my experience of working with a range of service users and carers, with local voluntary groups, lecturers and administrative and support staff. I will endeavour to highlight key events within a journey which stretches over a five-year period. I will utilise the five levels within the ladder of involvement outlined by Goss and Miller (1995) as a framework to illustrate progression within the School (more discussion of the ladder of involvement is given in Chapter 1). I will attempt to provide examples of the challenges to me as a manager, and how I used my role to influence, facilitate and support the enhancement of service user and carer involvement. The chapter gives practical examples of work undertaken to provide the readers with information which may be helpful in their own setting. These are offered as a set of possible approaches based on a specific set of experiences, rather than as a template.

7.2   Background Information

I was appointed at the university in 2002, initially as Divisional Leader for mental health, with responsibility for a team of mental health lecturers and a growing portfolio of undergraduate and postgraduate mental health focused courses, for nurses and other healthcare professionals. I soon became aware that there was limited input from service users and carers into these courses. Involvement appeared to occur through piecemeal arrangements across a small number of courses within the School, usually where lecturers had personal links with local voluntary groups and specialist services. Within a few months of my appointment, I made an effort to meet with coordinators of some of the local mental health groups to try to understand how best to work with their members.

All divisional leaders within the school had lead responsibilities linked with being part of the School executive team. I was subsequently asked to lead service user involvement, since there was a recognised need for someone to champion this within the School. I was aware at the time that my peers assumed that, because I had a background in mental health nursing and psychological therapies, I was more experienced in this area. While this was marginally true, it was a risky assumption to make. I feel that I was only slightly more knowledgeable, and certainly no expert.

Fortunately, at this time I was able to join a national steering group based at the Northern Centre for Mental Health, which developed a continuous quality improvement tool for mental health education and training course providers. Involvement in the development of a self-assessment tool enabled course leaders to measure levels of service user and carer involvement. The School became involved in a pilot study of the self-assessment tool. This provided staff with a development opportunity that was extremely valuable while expertise in this area was still emerging (Northern Centre for Mental Health, 2003). On reflection, I feel I was prepared to challenge others for the benefit of good practice, supported by a strong belief in equality and human rights. I was aware at the time of being willing to learn and grow with others involved. This helped me personally to progress and to lead the School on a journey climbing the ladder of involvement, overcoming a series of obstacles along the way (Goss and Miller, 1995).

In September 2004 I assumed a new role as Associate Head in the School, with a broadening of responsibilities, including operational day-to-day management in the School and line management of divisional leaders and, ultimately, a large number of academic staff. The role afforded me with a privileged position of contributing to School and Faculty strategies and policies, with access to senior managers across the Faculty and University. This proved instrumental in placing me in a pivotal position to facilitate others. Developments proposed by lecturers and service users could be directly put to senior staff, since I had membership of various School, Faculty and University committees. I feel that I have been able to open doors for service users, carers and lecturers by acting as their advocate.

I will now illustrate this, summarising the sequence of events using the ladder of involvement.

7.3 Level One: No Involvement

In February 2004, the process began by convening a School service user steering group with the purpose of enhancing the level of service user involvement across all courses (Box 7.1).

Box 7.1 Purpose of the School Steering Group

- To provide a forum fostering partnership working between academic staff and representatives from local service user/carer groups.
- To integrate a service user/carer perspective within course development, delivery and evaluation.
- To seek to ensure the achievement of the service user/carer statements and standards within the School of Nursing.
- Develop a guide for good practice for service user/carer involvement.
- To promote service/user carer involvement in aspects of research activity.
- To provide consultation on service user/carer perspectives for sub-working groups within the School of Nursing.
- To enhance networks between Comensus, local and regional service user/carer groups and course teams.

There was no existing explicit written Faculty or School strategy guiding staff to do this, although it could be argued that it was implicit within the learning and teaching and research strategies. Initially, I invited academic staff from across the School that had an interest or experience in this area. The Comensus initiative, with its extensive links into the local community, was able to assist in recruiting service users to this group. I was pleased by the response with steady growth in numbers attending, rising to sixteen by the third meeting, split evenly between lecturers and services users. I made it clear that the success of the group would be dependent on individual effort and contributions, all of which needed to be respected and valued equally amongst academic staff and service users. This appeared to be one of the most important principles to reinforce at each steering group meeting.

Terms of reference were written collaboratively by the group, initially focusing on service users and not carers. While the group recognised the need to include both, it was agreed that attempting to do everything all at once would create unrealistic expectations, heighten frustration and set ourselves up to fail. It was agreed that the term 'service user' be used as a generic term encompassing other terms such as patient, client, resident and public, while respecting differences in individual needs and terms used in different healthcare settings. The term selected reflected language used within our partner placement provider organisations. From the beginning, I had the benefit of administrative support for producing the agenda and minutes of meetings, updating records of steering group membership, maintaining information housed within a central data base, organising room bookings and refreshments and circulating documents. This proved to be an invaluable resource and contributed immensely to the progress of the work of the steering group.

The group initially met in alternate months. One of the first tasks on which the steering group agreed was to scope the level of service user involvement existing across the School, in an effort to determine the baseline from which to measure future progress. It emerged that there was anecdotal evidence that service users and carers were involved in some teaching in a limited number of modules. However, this appeared to be fragmented on an ad hoc basis, and very difficult to evidence at times of audits and during internal and external quality assurance monitoring visits. The scoping involved the administrative assistant requesting information from module leaders by e-mail and capturing what was returned, using a template grouping activity across divisions and courses. This eventually developed into a catalogue of good practice (termed a 'Good Practice Guide') occurring across the School, in an effort to share information with other divisional leaders and course leaders.

In the first academic year of the initiative (2004–2005), there were 48 examples of service user involvement listed, occurring in different modules. This might suggest that the School had already moved off the first 'no involvement' rung of the involvement ladder. However, there were many modules and courses with no service user or carer involvement, and some lecturers even questioned the need for such engagement. For example, in one conversation a lecturer who was in a senior position within the School stated that service users were the students, and, since student representatives were involved in providing feedback to course management committees, this sufficed. This, and similar conversations early in the life of the steering group, provided me and other fellow steering group members with an indication of the amount of work that needed to be undertaken. The new initiative provided a significant opportunity to challenge such myths and stereotypes.

Within the first year of the steering group it became clear that there was a high level of passion and commitment to the cause of engagement and of improving the student experience amongst individual lecturers and service users (Whittaker and Taylor, 2004). As understanding developed, there was acknowledgement of local and national drivers, which reinforced the work of the group. The United Kingdom review of mental health nursing in 1994 had been instrumental in advocating inclusion of patients in course delivery, seeing this as good practice (DH, 1994b). Academic staff within the School were very familiar with responding to national and regional policy documents, so I quickly learnt to present these at every opportunity to help articulate why service user involvement was important.

7.4   Limited Involvement

In February 2005, a year after the steering group was formed, its terms of reference were reviewed and amended to include a focus on enhancing carer involvement in the School. There were academic staff and carers who had been disappointed that this had not been included from the beginning, and some lecturers were already including relatives, partners and significant others to share their experiences with students. Unfortunately, this information had not been systematically recorded or promoted at the School level. At the steering group, some lecturers reported on their contacts with specialist groups and networks they attended including local service user and carer voluntary groups. Two mental health lecturers were, and still are, members of the executive committee of a regional voluntary mental health organisation, which provides support to service users and carers. Some lecturers reported how they had retained the contacts they had established while they had been in clinical practice, prior to working at the university. Others had actively sought out these groups with the intent of providing the students with the benefit of an alternative perspective from the clinical specialists who were also brought in as guest speakers. This appeared most evident amongst lecturers who were proactive when developing their module timetables, in the areas of mental health, learning disabilities and pain management.

In the second year of the steering group there was a fairly regular number of academic staff and representatives from service user and carer groups attending and contributing. They included the Faculty coordinator of the Comensus initiative. It was decided to formalise the roles and commitment people were making to enable staff to be recognised for their contribution. I requested that all divisional leaders provide me with the names of their divisional representative on the steering group. In some cases this led to two nominations being given so that attendance at meetings could be shared. This resulted in staff already involved being recognised by their peers in their respective division, as the divisional representative. In those divisions with no one attending a lecturer was nominated. A key part of my role was in motivating and valuing these representatives.

The School provided courses in pre- and post-registration nursing, operating department practice, paramedic practice, complementary therapy and psychological therapies, so, by virtue of the group sharing practice, we indirectly also promoted the interprofessional learning agenda. The plan was for these staff to support each other and act as 'academic champions', feeding information between the steering group and course and module leaders, and guiding others on how to enhance teaching, learning and assessment practice by involving service users and carers.

One of my responsibilities within the School was to annually update a number of its documents and handbooks. This included the manual written for staff and external visitors, and the handbook given to all new and returning students. In

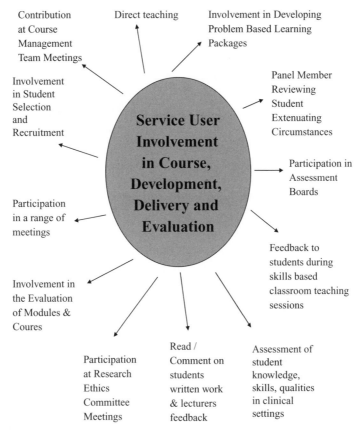

Contribution at Course Management Team Meetings

Direct teaching

Involvement in Developing Problem Based Learning Packages

Involvement in Student Selection and Recruitment

Panel Member Reviewing Student Extenuating Circumstances

Service User Involvement in Course, Development, Delivery and Evaluation

Participation in Assessment Boards

Participation in a range of meetings

Involvement in the Evaluation of Modules & Coures

Feedback to students during skills based classroom teaching sessions

Participation at Research Ethics Committee Meetings

Read / Comment on students written work & lecturers feedback

Assessment of student knowledge, skills, qualities in clinical settings

Figure 7.1 Long-term plan for service user involvement – School of Nursing, Faculty of Health, UCLan.

an effort to be more strategic, and to demonstrate that the School was committed to enhancing service user and carer involvement in course development, delivery and evaluation, an overall plan was developed by the steering group to articulate how this could be achieved through different activities. While this was written as a mission statement, it was also represented diagrammatically summarising examples of how service user and carer perspectives could be undertaken within course and School activities (Figure 7.1).

The steering group generated a desire to extend involvement beyond classroom teaching into School meetings. Since I chaired the School academic standards forum I was able to invite service users to attend and contribute. The forum focused on the enhancement of quality and standards and implementation of university academic regulations. School leads of working groups also reported on progress of their groups, and on the implications of changes in professional regulatory body standards for education. Needless to say, there were some challenging and productive discussions. It soon became apparent that having some consistency from a few service users who acted as the service user representative on this and other groups reduced the time I needed to undertake on briefing service users about the structure and terms of reference of the group and specific items on the agenda. Fortunately, the Comensus coordinator also attended, and assumed responsibility for briefing and debriefing service users.

Within the School plan, staff were encouraged to involve service users in divisional meetings. This has since occurred either as invitations for service users to attend specific meetings to discuss particular issues, or as regular attendees, such as has occurred at mental health division meetings. While it was an aspiration at the time, it was felt important that the steering group set out the vision of how service users and carers could be involved in areas such as research, module assessment, student recruitment and development of teaching and learning resources to name but a few. The strategy was crucial in guiding involvement within the School to another level.

7.5   Growing Involvement

In November 2005, the steering group reviewed the progress achieved by the group in relation to the terms of reference. The 'Good Practice Guides' were considered to be a particular achievement, capturing creative examples of service user and carer involvement across divisions and courses. It was agreed to be more systematic and update these at the end of each academic year, so that examples were coded by the year they were introduced. This enabled me, on behalf of the group, to include the guides in an annual report presented to the school executive team as evidence of achievement of the work of the steering group. The good practice guides were placed in a central database accessible by all academic staff, together with steering group minutes and all related documents. As other academic staff became intrigued by the work of the group they were able to access useful information.

Around this time lecturers, service users and carers came together with staff from other schools within the Faculty to share their experience and good practice. This appeared to boost confidence in many staff and encouraged them to submit abstracts for national and international conferences, resulting in verbal and poster presentations, thereby celebrating their efforts. There was evidence of a small number of staff involving service users and carers in writing learning and teaching packages for use with students. One mental health lecturer engaged in regular clinical practice through an honorary contract within a local mental health Trust and invited willing service users to share their experiences in an effort to ensure that a problem-based learning package for use with small groups of students was authentic and not contrived. The package was evaluated by students and staff, and amended accordingly. Effort was also made to feed back this information to the service users involved.

Similarly, a member of staff who wanted to share personal experience of blindness with nursing students, in the hope that this would help others, approached me. This centred on experiences in a local National Health Service Trust, highlighting what was good and what could have been improved in the way staff communicated. I met with this person and then through the School steering group we decided which course and module the experience would best fit, according to the module learning outcomes. The subsequent teaching session was videoed and included in the module Web CT (Web Course Tools) area for future groups of students to see. Key questions to aid facilitating discussion relating to the video were also drafted. This ensured that students were prompted to think around areas of practice which had been highlighted as important from the service user perspective. Both the development of the problem-based learning package and Web CT video were used as pilots within the School, and reported at the steering group for discussion.

This experience and parallel developments within Comensus led to recognition that we needed to develop a protocol which would guide staff when they wanted to develop learning and teaching resources (Appendix 8). Information leaflets and consent forms, which were forwarded to the School executive team, University solicitor and Faculty Ethics committee for approval, were devised within the group (a model consent form is shown in Appendix 9). This proved to be a very lengthy process. Eventually, by draft seven, the protocol and documentation was approved. It is now used across the School, and has been adopted by other schools. Service users were particularly helpful in amending the language used in the consent forms and information leaflets that explained how a person could help in developing the resource. Separate consent forms were developed for use with children and young people, with adults, and with individuals representing organisations. The inclusion of graphics made the forms more user friendly. The protocol highlights how long documentation and the resource is retained and where and with whom they can be used. A real challenge for me was acting as mediator between all groups involved, with the whole process taking almost two years to complete. A compromise had to be reached between the language typically used in formal university documents, and making them accessible to others, including service users and carers.

As the steering group matured it was felt that it would be helpful to everyone if case studies of involvement were shared as a standard item on the School steering group agenda. Representatives from each division rotated in asking staff to present, and the steering group gave feedback on good practice and areas for future improvement. I believe that the presentations served to enhance attendance at the steering group, assisted in maintaining standards, congratulated people for the work they were undertaking, and provided inspiration to staff. People started to send me information on useful resources available, including Web sites, commercially produced audio and video training resources and other interactive training packages. These were taken to the steering group to share with divisional representatives and disseminate to course and module leaders. The representatives would review the quality of the resources and feedback at future meetings. In turn, this fed into a list of relevant Web sites being archived on the central school database for all staff to access.

In my role I have responsibility for helping to shape the agenda for the two school staff conferences occurring each year, attended by over one hundred academic staff and researchers. The purpose of the conference is to provide an opportunity for staff to be updated on current developments and policy changes for implementation. Small group activities are often used to address emerging issues and devise solutions, sometimes through development of new procedures and protocols. I monopolised the afternoon of one of the conferences to promote the service user engagement initiative, together with other key staff committed to enhancing service user and carer involvement. Examples of good practice were shared with staff in a large group, which included positive feedback from students on how much they valued this experience. Academic staff were grouped in their respective divisions, consisting of approximately eight groups of between eight and fifteen staff. A structured activity involved them reviewing what they were currently doing and how they could enhance this, resulting in action plans to be achieved in the coming year. The 'academic champions' who contributed at the School steering group were central in this process.

Around this time, as a member of the Faculty Executive Team, I was appointed as Faculty lead for enhancing service user involvement in curriculum. While the School had a service user and carer steering group, faculty-wide user involvement was supported by the Comensus project. It was important to align the two initiatives, reducing duplication of responsibilities and maximising mutual support. The Comensus coordinator attends and contributes at a range of school and faculty meetings, to either update everyone on the work of Comensus or, along with a member from the team, to provide a service user perspective on what the group, forum or committee was doing. In addition, it was arranged for the Comensus coordinator to regularly be invited to the School executive team meetings. This enabled us to look critically at where things were working well, such as the courses where service users were involved, and where this was limited, so that action plans could be put in place.

These action plans were reinforced within the university internal quality enhancement process known as annual monitoring. This involves annual reports being written by module leaders, course leaders and divisional leaders which all feed sequentially through each other into the Head of School report written by myself on his behalf. By amending the templates used by all these staff, I was able to include a question asking that everyone report on the level of service user and carer involvement in modules and courses. Where this was acknowledged as limited, there was an expectation that this would be included in the next year action plan for enhancement of that module or course. In summary, academic staff were being asked to self evaluate their level of engagement with service users and carers, using a standardised university quality enhancement system. Over time, some staff used the ladder of involvement to self-assess their module or course, consciously recording as a team what level they were currently at, and what they could do to progress to the next level.

7.6 Collaboration

In November 2006, the Good Practice Guides for both service user and carer involvement were updated. They now extended to several pages long, showcasing examples of interesting and innovative practice. What was pleasing was that the guides were proving helpful in both internal and external quality assurance reviews and monitoring visits as evidence of innovation. The Quality Assurance Agency (QAA) major review audit provided a platform to showcase the totality of involvement initiatives, including the good practice guides and other documentation illustrating work of the steering group and the overarching support of Comensus (DH, 2003; Faculty of Health, 2005). Pleasingly, meetings with service users and carers were recognised as good practice within the School and Faculty and very progressive compared with other universities. Similarly, during a number of Nursing and Midwifery Council (NMC) approval and monitoring events the school received acknowledgement of good practice, recognising the strategic and systematic level of service user and carer involvement.

What was now evident was involvement of service users and carers at a variety of levels within the university from module, course and School level, and at Faculty and university level. This involvement could be described as occurring at micro, meso and macro levels. It seems to express a movement towards collaborative working, with increasing joint enterprise between service users and staff. Examples highlighted in steering group meetings included involvement in course development and validation events, teaching in large and small groups, providing feedback to students undertaking skills training, involvement in work of the School recruitment group, academic standards forum, divisional meetings and School executive team meetings. Admissions tutors for the pre-registration nursing course worked with service users in writing questions to be asked when interviewing prospective students. It was agreed that, with intakes of around 800 students annually, it was unrealistic to expect service users to be directly involved in all the necessary interviews.

Service users have since contributed at recruitment events including university open days to talk to prospective students. They have produced video clips demonstrating inclusion of service users and carers within courses that the potential recruits might study. These clips have been played while students are waiting in reception for their individual formal interview. They have also been placed on course and School Web sites. Service users have written questions to be included in students' clinical assessment documents for use by mentors and practice teachers when the student is on clinical placement. The documents request assessors to elicit and record service user and carers views of the student's level of competence and proficiency, enabling documentation of feedback first hand from the person at the centre of nursing care.

A further example of collaborative working is in the joint production of a DVD as part of an interactive education and training package aimed at enhancing knowledge and skills of primary care mental health practitioners. Service users and carers worked with lecturers to write the scenarios for the video clips to illustrate experiences of multidisciplinary team working, reception and consultation in primary care, clinical supervision and practitioner documentation (Harrison *et al.*, 2006). School staff and service users who worked with us were also engaged in the production of a CD-ROM resource, developed to support the national Primary Care Graduate Mental Health Worker (PCGMHW) programme. The input into the PCGMHW course was grounded in our close relationship with Preston Mental Health Service User Forum. This group reported later that when the first cohort of PCGMHW students completed the course and were taking up their posts with local General Practitioners, they began attending Forum meetings to continue these links and request that Forum members had involvement in planning and strategic development of their roles. This neatly squared the circle regarding people's desire to be part of something in the university that ultimately was of real influence in practice. It is pleasing that much of this experience has been shared by academic staff, service users and carers presenting jointly at national and international conferences.

United Kingdom policy advocating a patient centred and patient led National Health Service helped reinforce the purpose and work of the steering group (NHS Executive, 1999; DH, 2001b, 2002b). Local service providers appointed patient and public involvement leads and staff to co-ordinate these initiatives that then provided us with further key contacts within service provider organisations. Emerging policies were very useful for articulating to academic staff the national and regional directives and requirements (DH, 2004b, 2006b, 2006c; Skills for Health, 2006). The School steering group was able to use these policies to argue that involvement of service users and carers in the development, delivery and evaluation of courses, prepares students to work within care settings which had targets to be patient centred and patient led. This felt very contemporary and useful when marketing courses.

7.7 Partnerships

By November 2007, systems within the School appeared well embedded. They demonstrated clear open commitment to service user and carer involvement supported by a variety of documentation. A real step forward was involvement at a strategic level. As a member of Faculty Executive Team meetings discussing the Faculty learning and teaching strategy, I was able to act as an advocate, ensuring that service user and carer perspectives were included. Further consultation was welcomed and valued by the faculty executive team directly with the service user and carer advisory group. Service user and carer representatives are now members of a range of Faculty and School groups that focus on strategic and operational management issues.

While some people felt that it was important to have service users present in all meetings and areas of School and Faculty activity, it has since been recognised that, as well as being impractical, this would mean sitting through agenda items that are less relevant. By targeted involvement, service users and carers have been engaged as 'consultants', drawing on their specific expertise in the same way as other specialists are utilised within the School. This requires mutual trust and respect. There is now evidence of working jointly with service users in broader aspects of academic practice including assessment of students (Duxbury and Ramsdale, 2007).

The School is now targeting requests for help from local services user and carer groups and the Faculty advisory group in divisions and courses requiring help to network with local groups. Those divisions and courses under-represented in the School good practice guides are now a focus, recognising that there is a continuous need to reappraise whether existing approaches to service user involvement could be improved, taking account of changes in healthcare delivery and issues that arise from this. There is now an expectation that module leaders negotiate the content and methods of delivery to be used with service users and carers. It is acknowledged that there are modules which lend themselves less well to service user and carer involvement, such as the teaching of anatomy and physiology and other factual subject areas. However, where possible, the template used for academic staff objectives linked with their annual appraisal includes their progress towards maximum engagement.

More recently, following university restructuring working towards devolved responsibility at School level, the Faculty Comensus coordinator is now based within the School reporting to myself whilst maintaining a Faculty-wide remit for the work. This has enabled a review of the groups existing at Faculty and School level and resulted in the merging of the School steering group and Faculty group into a new advisory group, while retaining representation from all divisions in the school, but widened out for similar representation from other schools. Having led service user and carer involvement for five years in the school, it seemed timely to hand this over to the Comensus coordinator. Perhaps a sign of true collaboration was how easy this was to do. While I continue to act as a support and guide, my role is now more facilitative and appears a true indicator of the progress that has been achieved.

Funding for students, course development and delivery comes from a variety of sources in health and social care, including the Higher Education Funding Council for England (HEFCE), regional National Health Service commissioners and service level agreements with local service providers. Recently the School housed a regional event bringing together representatives from commissioners, service providers and various disciplines of academic staff from neighbouring universities. The purpose of the event was to share existing good practice, and to develop principles for commissioning, including performance statements and standards for service user and carer involvement in education.

While it is up to universities to fulfil the requirements of contracts by allocation of resources according to course need and professional body requirements, service user and carer involvement has typically be seen as implicit within this and viewed as good practice (Health Life Sciences Partnership, 2008). The Faculty and School have funded support for service user and carer involvement for a number of years, acknowledging that in order to prepare staff to work within patient centred and patient led services it is important to integrate involvement throughout the pre- and post-registration portfolio. One view may be to ring-fence money for this, while others may prefer some flexibility in how and where to allocate such funding to enable creativity. It is pleasing to see that commissioners are now considering this within contracts. Involving the service users who are our colleagues in such discussions appears to be the ultimate in partnership working.

7.8   Conclusions

My role has evolved over a number of years. At times I have acted as an ally, advocate and supporter for Comensus to ensure service user voices are considered. At other times I have led, guided, mediated, facilitated, challenged and supported a range of academic staff, service users and carers within the School, Faculty and University. Ultimately, however, this has been a journey of mutual learning and discovery, reflecting the spirit of partnership for which we have been collectively striving.

Service uses and carers have been actively involved in different aspects of the operational day to day issues within the School, to ensure the service user and carer agenda is realised. Service user and carer perspectives have also influenced School and Faculty strategies, policies and procedures in a myriad of ways. Any limits to the extensiveness of this involvement reflect key structural issues, such as availability of resources including time, expertise and dedicated funding.

The involvement activity within the School has progressed along the ladder of involvement supported by service users and carers, academic staff, and administrative staff. At one School steering group review meeting the ladder of involvement (Goss and Miller, 1995) was reflected on in terms of its value for school-wide evaluation of progress. The linear and hierarchical dimensions of the tool should be acknowledged and not applied in an overly simplistic manner. For instance, some staff felt judged when labelled at different points on the ladder; a consideration which needs to be respected and handled sensitively. By viewing the process within a broader commitment to continuity, development and systems, progress is not finished if partnership is reached in one specific area of the university. Similarly, we have used the five levels of the ladder for awareness-raising, not as a tool to point out failings. It has been used to self-evaluate at module, course and School level as a means to develop actions plans for enhancement, thereby sharing ownership. Rather than climbing the ladder of involvement to the top and stopping, we continue to strive for progress and as comprehensive an extension of involvement as we can manage across all aspects of our work. We acknowledge that this is a continuous process, which requires funding, support and commitment by individuals at all levels within the organisation.

8 Stories of Engagement

Helping influence nurses is very rewarding and one day you may be nursed by a friend, instead of just a nurse.

8.1 Introduction

This chapter comprises personal narratives from people associated with service user and carer participation in universities. Voices come from those directly involved with Comensus and from other United Kingdom universities and wider networks of support which have supported our work.

8.2 Service User Voices

Comensus has at its core a strong volunteer base, committed to engagement across all levels and striving for authenticity in all of their endeavours. The following are the voices are those of members who give so much to the project in the Community Involvement Team (CIT, the service user and carer led forum attached to Comensus) and from the wider community affiliated to the initiative. All of these individuals have been thoroughly involved in the work of the university, typically in a teaching role, but also in the development of teaching provision, research activity, strategic input and community liaison. Some of these participants have become involved relatively recently; others have been active in community groups linked to the university before Comensus was established and were intimately involved in setting up the project.

8.2.1 Keith Holt

The first meeting of what is now Comensus was held at the Gujarat Hindu Centre, Preston, in 2004. The idea proposed was for the University of Central Lancashire (UCLan) to engage the community in teaching and learning, thereby raising awareness of difference and disability, a unique innovation, an unknown challenge. At this embryonic stage, involvement was being offered to those living within Preston. On reflection, to start at a local level seemed sensible to test whether interest in involvement was present; however, this did not reflect UCLan's student catchment area. Unfortunately, I did not reside within the catchment area and did not have the opportunity to get involved in the CIT until 2008.

In 2008 I was interviewed by my peers, the already established members of Comensus, and was accepted to the main working group. I had had previous experience of engaging with the University, as I was a current member of Giving Experience Meaning, a group of mental health expert-by-experience trainers who train health and social care professionals and raise awareness of mental health and help stamp out stigma. Our experiences within the university had been positive, especially from those embarking on careers in health and social care services.

Joining Comensus built upon these experiences and allowed me to use skills I had learnt from being a member of the Service User and Carer Advisory Group (SUCAG) attached to the social work department, also based here at UCLan. Being a member of Comensus has led to my engagement in a wide variety of involvement opportunities and a greater insight into the everyday running of a university. Meeting so many people, Comensus members, community members, tutors and researchers whose genuine commitment to the concept of community involvement and improvement of practice has been outstanding, has benefited me enormously, raising my confidence and self esteem, and at the same time giving me the opportunity to put something back into services.

Recognition must be given to those 'Champions for Change' who recognised the need to empower service users and carers and enable them to get involved. Here everyone is a stakeholder. Logically, higher education is the place to promote and to give people the practical skills to work in partnership, ensuring that services provide person centred quality services.

8.2.2 Carol Catterall-Maguire

I led what might be considered a busy but relatively normal life until in my forties. I was unaware that I had the genetically inherited connective tissue disorder Pseudoxanthoma Elasticum (PXE). Although I had experienced various symptoms of this condition for over thirty years, it was the damage to my eyes that brought me to diagnosis. In January 1999 I was finally diagnosed and, in December 1999, my sight had deteriorated to the point where I was certificated and registered as blind. Worsening vision had made it no longer safe to continue driving a car or carrying out the duties of my profession – a neo-natal nurse – or be able to fulfil my role as a further education lecturer. It was at this point that I joined the ranks of the disabled and my life and societal standing changed irrevocably – or so it felt.

Comensus has given me the opportunity to express my feelings and experiences to those who provide or will provide for the needs of those who are incapacitated or fall into the group considered 'disabled' by wider society.

For me, being part of Comensus and speaking of my experiences gives me a sense of empowerment that comes from sharing my knowledge. For students, this leads to understanding and awareness of individuality in real life terms. My involvement can also lead to the needs of other service users being satisfied now and in the future.

8.2.3   Jacqui Vella

I am alive and it feels good. When Comensus was in its infancy I was the Chair of the Patient and Public Involvement Forum (PPI) for Lancashire Teaching Hospitals. I help run a diabetic support group and I was, and still am, the Chairperson for Breathe Easy, Preston.

The PPI told me about Comensus and I thought it would be too political, so I put it out of my mind. Then a friend telephoned me and asked if I would accompany her to the first meeting in the Foster Building at UCLan, so I decided to go along. I think someone mentioned snacks. I have always thought that universities were far out of reach and it would probably be over my head. I found instead a warm reception and a group of like-minded people who also wanted to give something back to services.

In my life I have had so much medical care and on many occasion been brought back from the brink through the care that I received. I joined the PPI after the sudden death of my husband. When I lost him my world fell apart. I had a heart attack, small strokes and started with diabetes. It seemed that anything that could drop off did. I had to retire medically from my position as senior accounts manager and I felt I would never get over being alone, losing my husband, my health and then, through illness, my income.

Back to the plot as I was telling you, I reluctantly went to the first meeting held to recruit new members for Comensus and I found warm friendly people who felt as passionate as I do about wanting to make a difference to the National Health Service. Little did I know then that it would become central to lots of things in my life.

My involvement with healthcare was quite wide through my work with the PPI and my hospital admissions. I could see the National Health Service with all its warts, but more importantly I could see dedication and compassion and the ability to rebuild the lives of the people who came through the doors. UCLan opened the doors to real opportunities to help nurses and social workers to see the importance of the things they do and how even the smallest things can help save a life or even, on the other hand, end it through minute things like not washing their hands.

My first encounter with students was so terrifying that I put so much Bach Rescue remedy on that I swear I was almost drunk. However, after 2–3 weeks I lost all fear and became a bit like wonder woman; nothing fazed me. Comensus is like a whole new universe. After my strokes I lost a great deal of ability and, although I never expected it to, Comensus gave me lots of skills and confidence that I had lost. I helped occasionally in the office with filing or sometimes using the computer to type, it all helped me remember words and skills but, more importantly, I was surrounded with new friends who like myself had been challenged by life, and we were all cheerfully sharing and learning.

Comensus is one of the most diverse groups I have ever belonged to: it is so multifaceted. Over the years that I have been involved we have all grown and learnt many new things. We share sadness and laughter. We are nurtured by the staff and they have enabled us to see our strengths and given us the courage to try new things. I am never afraid of looking silly or think I cannot do it, as their response is to help us develop and sustain us.

If more people stood back and looked at the ever changing face of the health service I am sure they too would want the privilege of being a tiny piece of building its future. I feel very blessed and thank the team for letting me take part.

I never dreamt that I could facilitate at a conference or help write new modules. A little piece of me wishes I had found all this intellectual stimulation earlier, as I might even have been a student. You never know in life what is next but I do know that I embrace each new day. I am not a bit political as a person but the National Health Service belongs to everyone, and universities, by involving patients and carers in their teaching of healthcare students, really do practise the government's vision of everyone having a voice. Things can only go from strength to strength.

8.2.4   Graham M Hough – Road to Comensus

I have been sectioned under the Mental Health Act three times due to my collecting lots of things at home and getting into trouble with the Environmental Health Department. After my last sectioned stay in hospital I saw an advertisement for service users to become part of a service user research committee that would ultimately review upcoming research projects in the National Health Service. I had already gained psychology and other health qualifications and fitted the bill. I was accepted on to the committee. A worker at a local mental health service user forum told me about Comensus and thought I might be interested.

I have been involved with Comensus since January 2008, going to meetings, helping to write social work lesson plans and have been involved in teaching these to postgraduate social work students. I have also been involved in a film festival devoted to mental health issues, where I gave a short presentation of my experiences of phobias and obsessive compulsive disorder, which health professionals and service users seemed to find enlightening.

I think Comensus is a very important new development in health education and should be encouraged throughout the higher education system across the country.

8.2.5   Robert Hopkins

I got involved in service user and carer involvement by encouragement from an organization that I was already involved in. I was doing voluntary work at Preston Disability Information Services Centre. One day the Volunteer Coordinator advised me that the University of Central Lancashire's Faculty of Health was setting up the Comensus Project, and they wanted to know what service users thought of the idea. I was encouraged to go along to the initial meeting at the Gujarat Hindu Society in Preston, in April 2004.

After that day was over a report of the proceedings was produced, then I was invited to a meeting with the late Eileen Johnson, the then Comensus Project Coordinator in the summer of 2004, to discuss the setting up of a Community Involvement Team (CIT). Then, at the beginning of 2005, I was sent a letter encouraging me to apply for the team. At first I was reluctant because I was not sure what I was letting myself in for. I received follow-up communications asking why I had not sent the form back. I eventually applied. I have never looked back since I was successfully appointed to the CIT.

I attended the first year's meetings, which consisted of administration and the setting up of the group. I found this was not very interesting. What did not help was that Eileen Johnson passed away in a road accident and there was no proper coordinator until Lisa Malihi-Shoja was appointed later in 2005. That was when the group started to get into the swing of things. However, gradually I got to meet people in the group and build a spirit of solidarity, comradeship and friendship.

What I like about the Community Involvement Team is its non-hierarchical structure; everyone has decision making powers. It is run for and by service users and carers.

Once that first year was over we got into the fun aspects of being actively engaged in teaching, training and research within the Faculty of Health. The highlight for me was when I took part in a couple of sessions of teaching first year nursing students on the learning disability pathway about Dyspraxia, the condition of which I am diagnosed. I enjoyed the big audiences (circa 500+ students). My feelings were of a rock star in that lecture theatre with that microphone.

My style in service user perspective teaching is all about using psychological methods, some of my colleagues on the CIT adopt different styles in accordance with their personalities. What I mean by psychological methods is all about getting the audience (the students) to remember what was said and to change their behaviours accordingly.

In addition, I believe in a Shakespearean approach to teaching, 'All the world's a stage and all the men are merely players, they have their exits and their entrances'. This means that everyone is an actor. I adopt this approach in my teaching in respect that all my lectures are theatrical performances. My performances have been hailed 'as one of the best teaching sessions ever encountered within the University'.

Other sessions delivered have included social work congresses and sessions to mental health nurses. The project allows me to meet and speak to well known members of the public, such as Sir Tom Finney, a well known footballer and carer who is our patron. Recently, I helped present service user led research at two international conferences: the first a social movements conference in Manchester; the second, our own conference, titled 'Authenticity to Action', in Grange over Sands.

More recently, we had to recruit more members to our successful team. I was on the selection panel. Our new members are diverse, which is proving a learning curve for me, as I did not previously have any contact with some sectors of society.

In summary, I feel that I and other members of the Community Involvement Team have gone from strength to strength. Long may it continue.

8.2.6   John Coxhead – Independence to Dependence

Going back to 1996, I enjoyed a healthy outdoor life as a landscape gardener and being self-employed made me a very independent person. However, overnight life changed that very independent person into a very dependant wheelchair user, now reliant on friends, and also made me find out who my real friends were. From a person using the car daily, to a person who sat looking at the car, unable to drive and relying on family and friends for transport.

I had no independence, when shopping, using public transport, or using any public services. In 1996 the wheelchair user was not recognised as an equal member in society but as the person in need of help or a burden on society. In 1996, at the same time as I lost my independence, the Disability Discrimination Act was introduced. Thankfully by now I had regained some of my independence by having a car adapted. Driving enabled me to join an access group. The group was made up of people with access or mobility problems.

The introduction of the Disability Discrimination Act gave people with access or mobility problems the power to force public and private service providers to make services accessible to the user experiencing problems. This access group gave me a feeling of value and that my dependence had been replaced by the chance to give people independence. At a meeting a colleague suggested I use my knowledge on access and mobility by joining a newly founded group, the Comensus project. I was not sure if this would turn out to be another name for an access group.

Attending the launch I soon discovered that Comensus was what I needed! A chance to get my voice heard and be taken seriously. I joined the Community Involvement Team (CIT) and discovered that working together as a team, a team that has personal experience on a wide number of disability issues, gives you a sense of belonging especially with the strength of the university behind us. The CIT gives people the feeling of value in that your ideas are being taken forward on how to train health professionals, including nurses and social workers. Thanks to Comensus and the way all CIT members are valued and how we are all treated as equals, people like me can once again begin to regain the feeling of independence.

8.2.7   Phyllis Prior-Egerton – What is it Like to Grow up With the Knowledge that You are Different, But Different to What?

I was closer to my sister than my brother. My sister was just one year older than me and my brother was five years younger. It was after my brother was born that I tried my first dress on, I felt great but guilty. I do not think I was aware why I felt guilty except it was my sister's dress. My dad was a vicar and my mum was involved in parish work, so sometimes I had the house to myself and took the advantage to get changed. When we moved from Wallasey to Weaverham in

Cheshire to a house with more rooms, 22 in all, they used to have jumble sales in the village hall. The jumble used to be stored at the vicarage in the outbuildings; guess who got the job of sorting it out!!! I could not wait for the house to be empty or my parents to be busy so I could try my new acquisitions on. Then guilt would rear its ugly head and I would rip them off. So, after some gardening, I would include the clothes on the bonfire. There used to be a jumble sale about once a month, so the process would then repeat itself.

There was one incident that happened in Wallasey which was scary. It was my first day at Somerville school, my mum had saved up to buy me a new coat specially for school; BIG mistake, I ended up bruised and battered with a new but ripped coat. That was my first and last day at that school.

Staying on the subject of school, when we moved to Weaverham I went to a private one in Northwich. Then I went to another one near Great Budworth. My grandfather paid for me to weekly board and my dad took lessons to help pay for school, too. So when, with all the sacrifice they are making, could you even think of telling anyone that my dad's star pupil and prefect is ordering you to go to bed with him in a dorm with other senior boys there.

When I left school I worked at a firm of agricultural engineers in Northwich. To get over my frustration, I used to ride my bike for miles and miles. I thought of asking my doctor for advice about the way I was feeling, but there always seemed to be a 'but': he was a friend of the family.

At this time there was nowhere to turn so you get on with life, get involved with work, meet girls, drive fast cars or, to be correct, drive old cars fast. Then the ultimate, get married, get your own business, get drunk, build up the business, get drunk. The business just happened to be a garage in the middle of Cheshire, near Tarporley. Included with the garage was a recovery business servicing the local transport industry with heavy vehicle recovery. Oh, nearly forgot, getting drunk to the state of only sober when drunk and 60 to 80 fags a day. O happy days hic, hic.

We now start the real decline – divorce, getting taken to the cleaners, not allowed to see my daughter. [Where is that bottle]. Problems again, where to live. So I convert the back of the garage into a room. Well, I had to have somewhere to sleep when I came in from the pub. I was still getting changed (female clothes) being Phyllis when I could. The trouble was still nowhere to turn, I was a bloke – so it said on the birth certificate.

I meet another girl/young lady and, yes, she gets pregnant, so yes we get married. This is it, I stop drinking – that is another story. New baby, new wife, the only trouble is I have drunk all the profits so have to sell the garage and my partner in the recovery business fiddles me.

There is only one way to go get on with life, buy a truck, go into haulage, as I have got a Heavy Goods Vehicle licence and have a certificate of professional competence. There is only one snag – Phyllis. There was another problem: my back, just as the business was picking up, all bills paid and money in the bank. Then bang, months off work then hospital. Nearly forgot divorce.

O well, start yet again, gets the truck on the road, find work. One or two false starts but managed to get some decent work. Then guess what, by accident I meet another woman and to save any misunderstanding tell her I am a transvestite;

even then I did not tell the truth. She seems to understand; this relationship lasted quite some time but I went back to my second wife. This did not last long, so my understanding lady came from Essex to live with me. We rented a house in Crewe. She had three children, two girls and a boy. She did not have a problem with me cross-dressing [O bliss]. We moved to North Wales nearer my main contract and I got another truck. One of the firms we were sub-contracted to went bust. Okay, so messed up again; one thing after the other, so I went bust. I started driving for an agency; good work, no worries, except for Phyllis. Otherwise things going okay, then haemorrhoids, went to doctor, red blood count under five, whoops into hospital quickly, five pints of blood.

I think it was about seventeen weeks off work. Then back to work for a small firm in Nantwich delivering pallets, a nice job going well – but bad luck again. I was delivering to a firm in the potteries, went in for breakfast sat on a faulty chair, whoops, not worked since.

I went for counselling re Phyllis, as she would not go back in her box; guess what – Tran Sexual not Tranvestite. So November 1996 living on own again, in a flat, as Phyllis. Due to the accident my appointment to Charing Cross, where I can have gender reassignment surgery, had to be cancelled but still on Premerin. A few months later an appointment was made for me to see a doctor at Glan Clwyd Hospital. She said she would take me on board but I would have to see a psychiatrist. I had my gender reassignment operation on 12 October 2000 but all sorts of things went wrong.

Whilst living in North Wales I had plenty of sexual harassment, crime committed against me and made to feel a freak and outsider. I now live in Freckleton and, through being a member of *Transinclusion* in Blackpool, I met the Comensus coordinator at one of the meetings and, after her very enlightening talk, I was invited to apply to attend an interview to join the CIT within Comensus. I was very pleased to be accepted. I have found the other members very committed bringing fresh dialogue to every meeting.

I would like to add that since I joined Comensus and, more importantly, since I was accepted on the Community Involvement Team, I have found that being involved with giving talks and getting involved with discussions with the students and members of the faculty at all levels has given me a sense of purpose in life. I hope that now I am able to give back to the community something that either groups or the individuals might find helpful. The other point I find fascinating about the CIT and Comensus is that we are all treated as individuals but together come together as a group, with a common aim in mind which is to improve things for future users of health services.

8.2.8   Russell Hogarth

I have been able to take part in lots of new experiences as a member of the Community Involvement Team at UCLan, and in lots of different ways, not just in teaching students. We also take part in and sit on advisory groups, steering groups; we are also part of the decision making process. We get involved in open days talking to students about life at UCLan and what we at Comensus can offer. We get involved in research projects too: we are taking part in a project called 'Bradton' with the University of Bradford. It is a project set on the Internet in the virtual world, where we have a town, a hospital and a university where people are virtual, not real, but the stories are factual. It is being set up to help students so that they can access it and find out all our life experiences whenever they want to. We are playing ourselves but changing our names and the names of the hospital and universities involved. Other on line projects include 'Sandbox'; we are hoping to help make the Internet work better for carers so that they will be able to access help easier.

I am enjoying my life at UCLan, meeting people and also making new friends and taking on new challenges. We are making a difference and helping to make improvements to healthcare practice.

I first came to UCLan for a meeting of service users and carers. It was at this that I first met Jacqui Vella, one of my colleagues at UCLan who mentioned the Comensus group. She told me all about the work they did speaking to students on health-related issues, and so on. I wanted to know more about it so I spoke to the coordinator and I was asked to attend an interview; something I had not done for forty years! I was accepted as a member; we have monthly meetings and the opportunity to speak to and teach students. We can go to lectures, film shows and attend disability group meetings. We also help out with teaching modules to nursing and social work students. We speak to all manner of nurses, theatre, accident and emergency, or very specialised ones; we tell them about our real life experiences and how even little things can make a difference to the patient.

I remember the first time I spoke to a class of students. I felt a bit nervous but I just related my story; it went well and I felt really good to be able to tell students what it was like to be looked after by nurses at some of the most vulnerable moments in my life. I always tell them the good things and the bad to give them the fuller picture, so that they can ask questions and reflect on how the bad things could be avoided and how good things, even little ones, be a really valuable outcome to comforting and sustaining a patient; best practice is highlighted.

After each training session, the students fill in evaluation forms which we can look at, as these help us to improve on how we teach future classes, as you can correct negative things and continue with the things that you find have helped. Students often say how they have benefited from the opportunity of talking to us and hearing our stories.

I have found UCLan a very friendly place and the staff are really lovely, and that is not just the Comensus ones. Throughout people are very helpful. We have disabled parking passes and library passes, which is great. We have comfort breaks built into each meeting. We also help each other. I read for a partially sighted member and, on occasion, she writes for me on the flipchart as I am dyslexic. Another member has problems seeing the screen if we are having a demonstration, so I am happy to read it for him. I have made many new friends at Comensus and we work really well together.

I had the opportunity recently to address the 2008 Nursing Conference in the Harrington Lecture Theatre attended by hundreds of students. I found it went very well due to the help I have received in training sessions on how to talk to students given by the Comensus team.

We have recently started taking and chairing some meetings of our own, without any university staff being present, and then reporting back to them for support.

The coordinator has been very patient and understanding with us, she comes out to our own charity groups to speak about Comensus so that the community can get involved. This adds a new tier to Comensus as we are now service users/carers and also the general community, which is very much in line with the Government's vision in health, everyone gets their say.

I feel our services at UCLan are well rewarded, not so much financially but in lots of other ways besides travel expenses and child care. We also have a lovely social dimension with away days and meals together. We all now feel a real part of the university and we are closely involved with the Faculty of Health and Social Care. We feel valued and know we can help make a real difference.

8.3 Peter Sullivan – Carer Involvement within the Faculty of Health at the University of Central Lancs

8.3.1 My Challenge

As a carer with a substantial caring role for eight years, why would I want to be involved with the Faculty of Health at the University of Central Lancashire?

I was approached by a lady who used to be a carers support officer but was now coordinator of the Comensus project looking for carers and service users for involvement at the university. I was aware from my involvement with other carers that there were two separate opportunities for carer involvement at UCLan, one with Comensus and one with the social work department called SUCAG (Service User and Carer Advisory Group). My main problem was of having enough time for involvement because of my caring role and as a carer working with many carers groups would I have the time? I went to the presentations/workshops to see if I liked Comensus and SUCAG and if they liked me. Strange that two involvement opportunities for carers in the same faculty arose at the same time. I was accepted on to both projects.

8.3.2 Involvement Opportunity Model One: SUCAG

Positives
- Introductory workshop attended by 70 mainly service users and carers who could further spread the message of service and carer involvement in social work education at UCLan. Issues discussed included:
  1. What do you want?
  2. What could you offer?
  3. What support do you need?
  4. Payment issues.
  Service users and carers selected for involvement got a boost from knowing that the net had been cast widely in the community.

- Department of Social Work only – valuable opportunity for me to spread the message of carers (especially young carers) to student social workers.
- Small group of three carers and three service users plus up to five academics (service users and carers in the majority). Good cross-section of carers and service users. Carers: parent carer, carer of a physically disabled person, carer of elderly person. Service users: disabled wheelchair user, ex mental health patient, ex drug and alchohol rehabilitation patient.
- Size of group enabled the group to move ahead quickly on interviewing and Congresses – day-long events addressing service user and carer perspectives for social work students.
- Size of group produced many opportunities, particularly if experienced in meetings, presentations, and so on.
- Opportunities to speak at three full day congresses per year to over 100 social work students on carer and service user issues.
- Opportunities on selection of students and to write 'think pieces' on carers, issues for the university Web site – so social work students can access information as and when required.
- Very positive approach to expenses, paying a realistic amount for attendance at meetings, selection of students and for teaching. Adaptable system so that service users and carers had the option to receive payment or donate to an organization of their choice.
- Environment issues addressed so that disabled service users and carers could contribute fully.
- Within two years felt that service user and carer involvement was an integral part of social work education at UCLan.

Negatives

- Lot of tension between academics, which sometimes spilled over into meetings, and a feeling that the service users and carers were under pressure to take sides.
- Because it was a small group with representatives lacking experience or confidence, more work fell on the few experienced, confident members. Not really successful in developing some members beyond attendance at meetings.
- Small intense group meant some service users and carers resigned as they felt unable to make contributions beyond attendance at meetings and possibly felt not contributing enough at meetings.
- Being a small group could not really 'carry' people while they developed their skills as it imposed more burdens on the other members.
- Time factor – felt under some pressure to volunteer for additional duties on behalf of group. Asked to represent carers on Departmental partnership committee on quality assurance. On this high-powered committee there was a hint of the token service user/carer.
- Lots of teething problems with the payments system that took the best part of two years to settle down.

- Support work largely fell on one academic, so when that person was away there was a problem with quorums. Actually did one Congress without support from academic staff.

Overall
- Great sense of achievement from the positive comments from the Congresses. Both written and oral comments and the individual one to ones who could relate to what we were saying. Comments like 'the best day of the year' and 'can we have more' make one feel that the input and difficulties, for example arranging care for the cared for is worthwhile.

8.3.3 Involvement Opportunity Model Two: Comensus

Positives
- 69 people mainly service users and carers came to the launch event. Three areas were considered in workshops:
  1. How should the 'community council' be involved in the Faculty of Health?
  2. How should the 'community council' be set up and run?
  3. How can we find out if the 'community council' is working?

  On the day 15 people expressed an interest in the involvement opportunity.
- The fact that the name of the group 'Community Involvement Team' came from the launch event gives one a feeling of ownership.
- Large committee of over 20 service users and carers.
- Very wide background of experience, ability and ethnicity.
- By apparently not turning anyone down there was a feeling that a very wide cross-section of carers and service users had been assembled.
- To overcome the dominance by a few, people round the table were asked if they had anything to say in turn; unfortunately, in some respect, this increased the pressure on the individual.
- As some people were struggling, there were debriefing sessions after the meetings to explore the tensions, problems and factors that restricted their involvement.
- Red and yellow cards were introduced to give everyone the opportunity to speak and to curtail the one or two who were dominating the meetings.
- The progress of some individuals can only be described as astonishing. Moving in a short space of time from not speaking and totally lacking confidence to making well thought out contributions that were appreciated by the other members. In time also moving on to delivering class room sessions.
- Numerous opportunities for involvement from teaching to ground-work for a social firm.
- In some respects, more of a personal development opportunity than straightforward service user and carer input to the Faculty.
- Very supportive of disabled members – accessible buildings, toilets, lifts, parking, and so on.

- Tremendous sense of achievement in producing a guide for accessible writing.
- Within three years to host and organise a three-day conference for carers, service users and academics from several countries represents unbelievable progress.

Negatives

- Large committee unmanageable in the early days. Big bang approach not planned, just evolved.
- There was no sense of being selected, as most people believed that everyone who expressed interest (and some others) were on the committee.
- Because of the diverse backgrounds from the wide trawl for members, there were people with baggage from the past which made cohesive working diffi-cult.
- Some members were very assertive and completely dominated others who simply never spoke.
- Some service users and carers had no idea of the extent of possible involve-ment. If they had they may have resigned. Some felt overwhelmed and did not contribute.
- Early meetings were the most challenging I have ever attended. After four hours only got to item two on the agenda. An observer said that this was a very poor use of my time and I should resign. I decided that my mission should be to stick with it and see if the meeting could be rescued. Use of post meeting debriefing, red and yellow cards and more assertive chairmanship pulled the meeting round.
- It appeared to me that very few of the service user members experienced any time constraints and were able to attend UCLan almost every day. This was very challenging, particularly for the carers who had extensive commitments. It was easy to feel that you were not contributing much.
- The monthly non-receipted expenses remuneration system was arranged at the lowest benefit level, that is, a low monthly figure that would not inter-fere with anyone's Income Support payments if it were to be interpreted as a payment. This was fine for people on Income Support but for regular attendees this had the appearance of receiving very little per hour. This was not helped by the more realistic payments made consistently under the other involvement opportunity.
- Also discovering at a later stage that honoraria for representatives from com-munity organizations attending advisory group meetings amounted to approx-imately 40% more for one meeting than the monthly expenses service users and carers got (albeit this was a payment to organizations, not individuals).
- The important issue here surrounding payments and expenses was that the complexities of trying to agree as fair a system as possible amongst a diverse group of people led to a feeling of unfairness in its application.

- Tendency for some service users and carers to become over possessive and resent any input from any other quarter. A refusal to accept that the university had interaction with individuals and groups in the community before this involvement opportunity.

8.3.4 Overall

Considering the tortuous beginnings, the fact that a successful three-day international conference could be held within three years is a fine testament to the commitment and ability of the service users and carers, and the support and encouragement provided by the Faculty of Health. On a personal note, I am pleased that I made the decision to stick with the involvement opportunity in the early days or I would never have seen or believed that a group of service users and carers could come so far.

As I was a carer on two different involvement projects in the same Faculty running parallel, I accept that I may see things differently from service users and carers who were on either of the individual involvement opportunities. It is impossible to consider one involvement opportunity without being influenced by the positives or negatives of the other project. In this account I have tried to show that some things went well from the start and some we had to work hard at to be successful. I feel that showing that we overcame hurdles and knock backs can be really useful to other people in a similar position, rather than give an impression that we all went to a meeting, came back and it was sugar and sweetness all the way.

8.4 The Advisory Group

Comensus has been very lucky that from its inception it has had a strong volunteer group – the Advisory Group which helps guide its work. This Advisory Group is made up of academics, members of third sector organizations and members from local statutory services.

8.4.1 Marie Mather – A Comensus Advisory Group Member's Perspective

The Comensus Project was formally launched in April 2004 and its existence was a key factor in my decision to take up a position at the University of Central Lancashire in January 2005. This service user, carer and community engagement action research study attempts to span the whole of the University Health and Social Care Faculty rather than to be piece-meal and ad hoc (Downe et al., 2007).

I view my journey as a new lecturer as inextricably linked to my journey with Comensus, which has enabled my growth in the delivery of joint lectures with service users and carers, effectively coupling the lived experience with theoretical underpinning ideas. I have built upon this to involve service users and carers in a strategic approach to developing the curriculum and in the promotion of good practice on an international basis through the presentation conference workshops.

I am an Advisory Group Member to Comensus and the continual access to service users and carers has broadened my perspective on teaching and enhanced student learning. I have been able to share that good practice with other institutions and learn about the different applications of involvement from them. This is my perception of what it entails to be an advisor to a group of service users and carers.

8.4.1.1   The Learning Curve: A Lecturer Perspective on Involvement

> Problem-posing education has dialogue as its vehicle, and dialogue requires direct involvement. (Bevis and Murray, 1990: 127)

Cannon and Newble (2000) posit that curriculum development be an ongoing process and can be guided by the expertise of many, including staff and students. A major learning experience for students is to be exposed to a variety of perspectives. The nursing profession and the development of student nurses should also be guided by the involvement of service users and carers.

Students can arrive in higher education with many preconceived ideas, skills and habits that have been learned throughout life. Some habits may be beneficial and some less useful (Race, 1999). While much emphasis may be placed on the acquisition of knowledge and skills, being fit for practice also involves the acquisition of appropriate attitudes. Rawlinson (1990: 116) explains the nature of personal attributes necessary to deliver client centred care:

> Consistent conscious awareness of the aspects of self within the nurse may enable or enhance the effective delivery of appropriate, considered, responsive, nursing interventions, which are sensitive, empathic and client centred.

Cannon and Newble (2000) refer to attitudinal objectives that require consideration of the views and opinions of others which may be different to their own. This is where the active involvement of service users and carers in our teaching can have a major impact on future nursing practice. Race and Brown (2001) talk about some lectures as deep 'life-changing performances'. The first hand and lived experience of service users and carers can effectively challenge and influence students in the development of their attitudes and their future nursing practice.

8.4.1.2   The Servant Teacher and the Servant Colleague

Robinson (2009) writes of a servant teacher as nurturing students to feel more comfortable, valued and supported, so that they can become the types of professionals who will not be content with the status quo and who will transform healthcare for the future. He states that this requires a re-examination of the use of power on the part of lecturers and developing an empathic listening approach while being available for students.

Adopting this nurturing role with colleagues is also equally important. The concept of the servant teacher can then be broadened to that of servant colleague. If the meaning of the term 'colleague' is examined within pedagogic literature, it generally refers to other academic staff: a narrow and misleading interpretation which ought to be extended to include service user and carer allies.

Realizing a shift in the balance of power in order to foster the development of fit-for-purpose students who will seek progressive change in nursing practice requires that we also need to affect a shift in the balance of power with service users and carers. All members of the Advisory Group, staff and service users alike, consider each other colleagues. Making a difference and influencing future nursing practice very obviously lies at the heart of my personal objectives and this is also central to the aspirations of those in receipt of care. As a servant colleague my responsibility is to help them to feel comfortable, valued and supported. I am confident that my colleagues in Comensus share this philosophy. They have certainly helped me to feel secure, valued and supported in this way. This creates a strong teaching and strategic development team.

Together we can foster and create an atmosphere of change within the attitudes of the future mental health nursing workforce. By giving access to a variety of perspectives and enabling student debate and discussion we can nurture each other and discover information together to promote personal growth and well-being (Robinson, 2009). Involving service users in true partnership will help the nurses of the future to meet the challenge of service user involvement in their own practice.

8.5 Staff Voices

Comensus is very fortunate in that it has a staff team comprising of a project coordinator and a part time administrative assistant, whose role probably exceeds the strict confines of administration extending into important aspects of facilitation and relational support. There are also a small number of academics who are closely involved and supportive of project activities, including one who shares office space with the project team. It is this staff team that facilitates the project and develops and supports all the members involved. The coordinator role is pivotal, and her story opens this section. Other lecturing and research staff either supports the project or makes use of it as a resource, and some of their stories are also included.

8.5.1 Lisa Malihi-Shoja – Project Coordinator

Being employed as a project coordinator for a service user and carer initiative is at times extremely difficult, at others extremely rewarding. One thing you never get to experience is boredom. The role places you in a position between two cultures – a 'no mans land'. You are neither an academic or a service user or carer, yet your role is to facilitate between parties and ensure a satisfactory outcome for all. Within Comensus we have been really lucky and had some fantastic academic champions who have supported our work and ensured we are included in activity. However, there are still pockets of 'resistance', academics who do not wish to engage with Comensus. They may not consciously be aware of this, but this oversight does sometimes mean our goal of systematic and inclusive engagement across the Faculty can be difficult to achieve. To overcome this we try to make ourselves indispensable, contributing to activity across the board; we sit on validation events, get involved in writing new modules, course programmes, input into Faculty strategy and engage in research and teaching. One of our members – Les Collier – used to say 'it is about winning hearts and minds' and this is the model we have used. We are constantly chipping away, celebrating our success, raising awareness, putting ourselves forward and becoming a part of the culture itself.

Becoming embedded into activity is our ultimate goal but for me this can raise all sorts of personal issues. I am employed to be the supportive voice for service user and carer involvement, yet I find myself becoming entrenched in the culture of academia. This is true also for our members. The more we sit on boards and meetings, the more we are aware of resource restrictions and I question whether we fight as hard now, as we did in the beginning, now that we are aware of some of the parameters within which we work. The converse of this is also true – as we are becoming more involved have we won these battles?

My past post involved supporting quite a radical mental health service user forum. Everything was a constant fight. Getting our voice heard was really difficult. We were either sidelined or, when asked to consult, not included authentically. This has not been my experience here. The Faculty does take service user and carer involvement seriously. Yes, it has not been easy, but at no time have we ever been marginalised. I can also honestly say that as an employee of the university I have never been told to restrict my involvement or comments; instead, our comments have been welcomed.

As a coordinator, getting help and guidance can be difficult. The main difficulty is that you do not have a blueprint to work off. Service user and carer engagement is relatively new to academia, with many models being implemented across the United Kindom and beyond. Each has its own difficulties and successes, but each differs from the rest in terms of funding, remit, resources and culture. The post itself can be very isolating. Part of it includes all the project management criteria, including budgets, writing reports, engaging in Faculty activities, writing bids, providing training, and so on. Part of it includes academic activities, supporting people to engage in teaching and research. Yet another part involves all the pastoral support for service users and carers, which sometimes can be difficult. The success of the project hinges on the service user and carer involvement, but sometimes people need extra support to engage. They may be going through life changes, diagnosed with illness, experiencing mental distress, lacking confidence, and so on. I do support and hopefully empower people to engage with us, but sometimes people need more than a phone call, they need you to listen to them, understand, empathise and support them through a difficult time. Some may question whether this is my remit. It is certainly not in my job description, but if we want a project built on kindness, support, engagement and understanding these are some of the things you undertake and undertake them gladly. I am very clear on boundaries and work well within them, but sometimes these become a little blurred. Recently a member of the CIT with whom I had built a long-term professional relationship died. The death hit me quite hard personally, yet my role is to support the group. It is at times like this when the role is particularly hard.

My role is for the most part very rewarding. We have lots of successes in many ways. I have been lucky enough to engage with extraordinary people who give so much. I have been privileged to see them grow in confidence and take on new and varied activities. I have seen the culture change (yes, it is slow but it is changing) and service users and carers populate the space in the university. We have been recognised by our peers for our good practice and innovative work. We have developed and expanded our work and remit. All of this is worthwhile when the students tell us that from listening to service users and carers they will make a change and try to improve services.

8.6 Service User Involvement in the Development of a Course

8.6.1 Joy Duxbury, Sue Ramsdale and Fiona Jones

For the Teaching Effective Aggression Management (TEAM) course, service users were part of a development team that also included academics, practitioners and service managers. In the early stages, the standard academic processes concerned with formally establishing and validating a course were a negative factor for everyone concerned, service users and clinical staff. Because of this, there was a concern that service user involvement might be rendered tokenistic. This was to alter significantly as we progressed the work and moved towards delivery of the course.

Initially, the student group (who were all qualified professionals) expressed a series of misgivings about the thought of service user involvement in this aspect of the course. The students' fears were allayed in discussions with tutorial staff, and many of the objections turned out actually to be grounded in an initial lack of clarity regarding expectations of the assessment process.

The format of the assessment, which took place over two days, involved student demonstrations of relevant skills based upon one pre-prepared scenario and one they were given to prepare and deliver on the day. Each student was given feedback from each panel member; there was also the facility for them to respond to this feedback. Given that many of the students had been wary of the service user involvement in the assessment process, their evaluations of the actual event were overwhelmingly positive. The panel was congratulated on giving convincing and constructive feedback. And the service user contributions were felt to be thought provoking and enlightening. Furthermore, one effect of the service user contribution to the process was a reported sense of increased confidence in working towards best practice. The latter point suggests to us that implicit in the students' experience of service user involvement was an enhancement to the validity of the learning process.

Service user participants felt that the process was tiring but they were gratified to note a positive effect for the students, connecting with wider hopes for improved practice once the students returned to the places they worked in.

8.6.1.1   Fiona Jones

Being involved as a service user assessor on the panel was brilliant. For me it was not just about assessment of the students, the chance to give feedback and talk about it is a way of teaching too. If you think about it, it is the way forward because who better to teach this subject than someone who has had these techniques performed on them? I found myself in a teaching role with the odd member of staff who had known me as a patient before. This was an important turn around for me and brought home how close the link is between training and making a difference in the real world. I got involved for this reason, to make sure nobody else detained in hospitals would have to go through what I went through. I got involved at the university because of links to the mental health forum where I had been volunteering and supporting the group. Once I had got involved, there was no stopping me. I have helped out on a number of courses and in developing new courses; I have also presented my experiences to large conferences of staff and students. I was invited to give a joint presentation with staff at an international conference in Canada, which was about secure mental health services. In the end I was unable to go, but I made a DVD to be shown, so that the conference still got to hear my point of view.

The insight that participating service users brought to this process from their own experiences added a unique richness and level of credibility to the process that could not have been achieved in their absence. Worries that this involvement could cause distress for participants proved to be unfounded. The overall module feedback from students unanimously requested that service user involvement should be thoroughly increased, and particularly taken up in the practical teaching of the physical training sessions.

8.6.2   Caroline Brown and Karen Wright – Lessening the Pain – Learning from the Voice of Recovery

It is a common adage that we 'learn from experience'. This is a story of learning from somebody else's experience. Academics and practitioners have sought various ways of giving real meaning to the learning process and to promote respect for clients of mental health services. Caroline has had significant personal experiences of mental distress and self-harm but is now in recovery; Karen has worked in relevant services and is now a university teacher of student practitioners who need to understand how best to care for people in such circumstances. In this teaching development we worked together to enrich student learning by bringing forward personal experiences into the classroom without the need for Caroline to be actually present. Instead, Caroline wrote a letter to the student group, and this was used in place of a more typical problem-based learning scenario. Thus *'problem-based learning'* became *'person-based learning'*:

Dear Nursing Students

This is my story. I trust you with this information. Please deal with it sensitively, as though I was asking you to care for me.

I changed schools when I was 13 and that was when my problems began. I felt that I was not as clever as those around me. This was really difficult for me because, in my family, a person's worth was judged by their academic success. Later that year I started harming myself – cutting, always cutting. I did not know why I did this – I didn't know anybody else that did it and I did not tell a soul. I cannot even remember the first time it happened, or where the idea came from to cope like this. Then throughout the next two years I just felt like shit and I drank a lot, particularly in the evenings after school. I would be with friends, but I would be the only one getting drunk. Then, when I got home, I would self-harm; it became a routine.

In the last year of high school I went to see my GP, I felt rubbish. He made me an appointment to see a counsellor at the surgery. I saw her twice and on the second time she discharged me because she said there was nothing wrong with me. (In actual fact, I hardly told her anything – I had told NO ONE about how I really felt and about my self-harming and was not going to start with her!) I didn't care…it is only now that I care.

I did my GCSEs, but did not get any 'As' – that was important and things got worse, at this stage I had felt that bad for two years. One night, at home, I tried to kill myself. I cut my wrists and went to bed. I was not expecting anybody; I did not expect to wake up, ever. My friend came around that night, she found me and told my mum – after that I went into a private hospital in Altringham (my family had private health care). I now think, looking back, they were in with a chance because I was at breaking point. But doctors do not get to know you as a person. I do not blame anybody…how does anybody see? How can they tell? I got worse in there – separated from everybody – and they did not make me feel any better. I got worse. I cut my arm so badly that I was lucky that they saved me and my arm. But the response was shock that I had deteriorated so quickly and they could still do nothing for me(!) and I was simply referred back to my GP.

In the January, I started seeing a NHS Community Psychiatric Nurse (CPN) weekly, at a Community Mental Health Team (CMHT) in town. Sometimes it was really hard because, for the first time, I was really saying how I felt rather than keeping it all in. I had more trust in her than the others and some times it went so well that I left feeling really good about myself. I got into college with her help and things went so well that I was discharged. That day I went to see my nana and walked down to the sea front. I felt real; I loved the smell of the sea and felt so good about myself. When I remember that day, I can still smell the sea. I did well at college and things seemed to be on the up.

Time passed, then for no apparent reason, I took a dip. The next time I saw that CPN was on the medical assessment unit after I had taken an overdose (she was on-call for A&E that day). Again I felt numb, I had no particular feelings about not succeeding at killing myself, I just did not want to be here any more and I when I felt like that, I felt too bad to tell anybody. I could not ring help lines or the services. I was cutting every day, usually at bedtime – those early hours of the morning are the loneliest.

So this is the first part of my story. It has been explained to me that this will help you work through issues that will be real in your practice, which is why I am happy to share with you my experience.

Things are very different for me now – but I will let you know about how that came about when you have had chance to think about what you would do, if you were responsible for my assessment and care.

Good luck

Caroline

This letter attempts to convey a very particular experience to provoke enquiry and learning for the student group. This required an honest and open reflection upon a time when the response of the nurse was vital to recovery. The student nurses approached this letter with the same organization and division of aspects of learning as they would do had it been a devised scenario written by the lecturer. The following week the students presented the work they had done and shared this with the rest of the group. Many different views existed as to what might have been the appropriate way forward in this case, and the management of the apparent risks. Caroline then wrote a second, follow-up letter to the students, seeking not to provide solutions but to provide some closure and a positive story of recovery, much of which was attained through effective working alliances and respect for her autonomy:

Dear Nursing Students

In my letter to you I tried to tell you about how I came to a point where I really needed mental health services to help me. You will be relieved to hear that help was provided and that because of this I was able to turn my life around. I started to see the same CPN again and she included, with my agreement, some other people in my care – a psychiatrist, an art therapist and a family therapist. The family therapy was not useful at all; the family were 'too far gone'. My parents have since split up.

I enjoyed the art therapy, and also a Cognitive Behavioural Therapy (CBT) assessment and therapy revealed that I was suffering from social phobia. This made a lot of sense because I really struggled with things like enrolling at college, ordering drinks at a bar, booking the car in for repairs, anything that needed me to communicate with people that I did not know. I had hampered my recovery in the past because I was too embarrassed to say what I was experiencing. I saw a psychiatrist, usually with my CPN, and had a number of medications, cipramil and trazadone being the main two.

Sessions with my CPN always left me with something to do (homework) and I always emerged with a feeling of being alive and energised. I knew that I had to get on with things. I even used to go home and tidy up. Every time I felt great – every time. Throughout my therapy with my CPN I never stopped cutting and she never asked me to. It was not the problem. She focused on me not my self-harming. Self-harming was not a problem to me. I could manage it and I also learned to manage my moods. These are some of the things she did:

- Got to know me
- Nurtured my trust
- Sometimes, if I was crying, she knew how important it was – she would sometimes let me cry and talk – but she knew when to tell me to get to work on the problem. I was not allowed to wallow in my sadness. I had to work at making things better
- We always looked at how I could change things by the end of the session – this was new to me. Everybody else had made me talk about how bad things were and then left me with that.
- Helped me with general life things, for example, enrolling at college, booking car in, making phone calls, things that made daily life possible and achievable
- Provided consistency
- Respected me
- I never felt like a burden or a time waster
- Never told me to stop cutting myself or made me feel bad about it
- Helped me to help myself when I had cut (gave me sterile dressings/ showed me how to put steri-strips on, and so on. (Also safer ways of cutting that were less damaging.)

Now I have not self-harmed for a year and I have just completed a degree in psychology – only having harmed myself about three times in the three years. I am a different person now – lots of things have made me who I am and obviously I have grown up too, but my self-harm was not about me being a child. It used to make me angry when people used to say 'you will grow out of it'. You never know, I may self-harm again – it's like a safety net. I have grown in maturity and health not because of the passing of time but because somebody helped me to grow through it.

Caroline.

One of the most interesting aspects of delivering this lesson can be the level of empathy shown by the group. Although Caroline is not there in person, the group discussions pivot on her very personal disclosure and the trust that is put in their capacity to treat her 'story' with respect. Professional carers have this privilege and responsibility every day, to see and respect the person and to hold their trust as a fragile and precious thing.

8.7 User and Carer Workers

The work of those involved in service user and carer involvement can be very isolating; as such, peers are very important. In the following section, Jill Anderson describes the work of the Developers of User and Carer Involvement in Education (DUCIE) and Chris Essen gives the perspective of a development worker at Leeds University. Both Jill and Chris have been effective allies of Comensus over the years, supporting ourselves and other similar initiatives throughout the United Kingdom.

8.7.1   Jill Anderson: Developers of User and Carer Involvement in Education (DUCIE)

Here the origins and evolution of the DUCIE network are described. A flavour is given of its work, and some information provided about associated involvement initiatives.

8.7.1.1   *Origins of the Network*

In the summer of 2005, a small band of service user and carer involvement development workers, based in universities, met over two days in Nottingham. They had in common that they were fairly newly appointed to posts set up to facilitate user and carer involvement in education for health and social care. Lively discussion was accompanied by a shared sense of optimism and enjoyment in the possibilities of these new roles. They were seen to pose significant challenges, too.

Asked to describe their roles, workers described:

- battling with confusion
- juggling too many balls
- spinning plates
- wearing lots of different hats
- working with different voices
- standing on tiptoes.

They spoke of being:

- surrounded by question marks
- in a fog
- wheeled out
- pulled in different directions at once
- parachuted in to rubber stamp things
- about to be rained upon.

The Developers of User and Carer Involvement in Education (DUCIE) network evolved from that first Nottingham meeting. Supported by the Mental Health in Higher Education (mhhe) project, but with a remit that goes beyond mental health, DUCIE has continued to meet three times a year. The network has the following objectives:

- To provide support, and meet the needs for continuing professional development, of involvement workers employed in universities.
- To share and disseminate good practice and examples of existing posts and initiatives.
- To provide opportunities for debate and the teasing out of complex areas of practice.

- To develop good practice guidelines.
- To act as a central point of contact for national initiatives, such as the Mental Health in Higher Education project, seeking to engage with users and carers involved in learning and teaching in higher education.
- To act as a campaigning and pressure group.

DUCIE meetings generally follow a similar format, with opportunities both to offer and to seek support. Informal discussion in the morning – information sharing and a round of 'current issues and challenges' – is followed by more structured discussion of key issues in the afternoon. Meetings function in a variety of ways.

8.7.1.2   Exploring Common Issues

There are differences between individuals, roles and settings but a lot of common ground:

Tokenism: User and carer involvement workers report being asked to find 'a user representative' for a meeting due to take place in two hours time – or, worse still, to be that representative. Lip-service can be a problem: In universities 'people say "Yes! Yes! Yes! Yes!" but they mean "No"'.
Differing priorities: This can lead to insecurity. 'Academics may be more interested to get a publication out of an initiative than to keep it going'.
Conflicts of loyalties: 'It can be difficult to maintain faith with the community members you are working with without alienating colleagues within the Higher Education Institute (HEI)'.

8.7.1.3   Identifying Patterns

It has been recognised, for example, that:

- User involvement initiatives in higher education often begin with something of a 'scattergun' approach (to get a range of activities established quickly), with the emphasis on quality developing over time.
- Progress may not be strictly incremental – universities which were ahead of the field some time ago, may fall behind as others 'leapfrog' over them. Restructuring can result in set-backs as well as progress in user-involvement initiatives.

8.7.1.4   Bringing Gaps to Light

A request for examples of university-wide involvement initiatives at one DUCIE meeting elicited no response. This seems to be the picture UK-wide: that different parts of a single institution act in isolation, with separate funding streams for education in the areas of health and social care. The resources of existing projects/individuals are often under-used and frequently not built upon.

8.7.1.5   Exchanging Solutions and Successful Strategies

When a DUCIE member spoke about lack of training opportunities, others spoke about how they had set about obtaining funding for – in one case – a part-time PhD. Examples from one institution can be used to achieve leverage in another.

When one member spoke about her lack of career progression, another detailed how his line manager had gathered evidence – from within and outside the university – to make the case for his promotion.

In one institution, where commitment of staff seemed to be wavering, a user development worker found an ally in the external examiner who was able to ask informed and incisive questions during programme reviews.

8.7.1.6   Sharing and Developing Good Practice

DUCIE members frequently share policies (for example recently, on the reimbursement of childcare and replacement carers' costs). They comment on one another's documents and strategies and have been involved in developing guidelines themselves – for example, on the employment of user and carer involvement development workers in Higher Education Institutes. Ethical issues (such as concerns around diversity or consent) are frequently debated. New innovations can be shared – the payment of a monthly stipend to all service users involved at one university for example; the instigation of a student award for involvement at another.

8.7.1.7   Debating Alternative Models and Approaches

DUCIE members challenge one another's notion about 'right' ways of doing things.

Not having a development worker can, for example, have benefits in terms of 'buy-in' from the whole department – staff cannot 'hive-off' responsibility to a single worker.

Sharing a room with academic staff can combat isolation, but has disadvantages in other ways (lack of privacy and space).

8.7.1.8   Lobbying

DUCIE members wrote a letter to the National Director for Patients and the Public, raising concerns about payment issues for service users in receipt of benefits.

8.7.1.9   Providing and Receiving Support

Support goes beyond the sharing of strategies and solutions. It is conveyed by a word or a gesture or a smile. DUCIE meetings provide an opportunity to 'let off steam' – to express feelings of anxiety, rejection or frustration:

Sometimes, when people are talking about the future, I wonder 'will I be here?'

I see what is happening elsewhere and people are discussing things together, but I am this kind of 'thing' that hot desks and no-one knows I'm there.

Staff say "service users need support". I say, "I'm a service user". They say "We do not think of you as a service user because you cope".

Meetings help to keep people going. They are not badged as such, but can function as 'peer supervision', in the absence of – or complementary to – locally based sources of support.

8.7.1.10   Seeking and Offering Recognition

It can be difficult to get recognition within one's own institution. Feedback from fellow DUCIE members can be useful in achieving this. Details of the Ian Light Award scheme – one tangible source of external validation for DUCIE members' work – are given in Box 8.1.

Importantly, the DUCIE network provides support not only to people appointed to user and carer development roles from outside the institution, but also to those staff members assigned to develop structures from within. Meetings are not about 'them' and 'us' – 'involvement workers' and 'academics' – and are open to all those willing to offer and receive support.

8.7.1.11   Evaluation and Linked Initiatives

Some light is shed on DUCIE by interviews and questionnaires from a recent evaluation of mental health in higher education:

DUCIE meetings ... have been incredibly useful, inspirational and helpful personally and have had a direct impact on taking my work forward.

DUCIE sets 'a very supportive challenge against the dangers of being complacent, or of thinking things are not possible'. It provides 'the opportunity to share vast amounts of experience and knowledge which is not available in books or courses'.

DUCIE is 'a great resource and has helped our project enormously'.

It is 'a great source of personal support and mainstay of the national involvement in education scene'.

DUCIE is an 'excellent network' which 'recharges my involvement batteries'. This person valued 'collaborative working with a range of people' and membership of an 'enthusiastic, committed network'.

DUCIE was initiated and has been sustained through the commitment and enthusiasm of its members. It draws strength from continuity, but also from a membership that evolves. It exists in a mutually supportive relationship with other projects and activities, including the Mental Health in Higher Education Project, the Ian Light Award for Work in Pairs and the Professional Education Public Involvement Network (Box 8.1).

> **Box 8.1**   Supportive Resources and Organizations
>
> *(i) The Mental Health in Higher Education Project*
> *Mental Health in Higher Education* aims to increase networking and the sharing of approaches to learning and teaching about mental health across the disciplines in United Kingdom higher education. Service user and carer involvement in education has been one key aspect of the project's work, which included joint development of *'Learning from Experience: Involving Service Users and Carers in Mental Health Education and Training'* (Tew, Gell and Foster, 2004). The project has a Web site, produces a regular e-bulletin and runs events and workshops (www.mhhe.heacademy.ac.uk).
>
> *(ii) The Ian Light Award for Work in Pairs*
> The late Ian Light, service user consultant and lecturer in health and social care at City University, was a founder member of the DUCIE network. This award, in Ian's name, aims to support and nurture user and carer involvement development workers employed in United Kingdom higher education, enhancing their effectiveness and capacity to effect change. It is organised by the Mental Health in Higher Education Project, the Centre of Excellence in Interdisciplinary Mental Health at Birmingham University, City University London and the East London National Health Service Trust. Further details can be found on the Mental Health in Higher Education Web site: www.mhhe.heacademy.ac.uk/ian_light_award.
>
> *(iii) The Professional Education Public Involvement Network (PEPIN)*
> PEPIN aims to share information and promote discussion relevant to the inclusion of patient, service user and carer voices in professional education. It is supported by an online forum. To date, this has been used to raise awareness of new initiatives, share resources and ask questions about thorny issues, such as payment and accreditation for service user trainers. It is open to anyone with an interest in the area, and benefits greatly from the contributions of users and carers involved in education and training. PEPIN's development was supported by the Medicine, Dentistry and Veterinary Medicine subject centre of the Higher Education Academy. It complements the work of the DUCIE network, extending networking to a broader community of practice. (http://pepin-uk.net/)

8.7.2   Chris Essen, Leeds University Service User and Carer Involvement Worker

I began working as a full-time Service User and Carer Involvement Development Worker in January 2005. The School had already established a written strategy document with the broad aim ensuring that service users and carers be involved as much as possible in all aspects of healthcare education and research. A Strategy Implementation Group (SIG) made up of School teaching staff, but with some service user representation, was charged with meeting this aim. It had recently appointed an Academic Lead for Involvement; based on his experience of progressing this work in mental health nurse education.

Although the strategy notionally covered research, we were directed by the SIG to focus on learning and teaching. The School is a large one, covering a number of healthcare disciplines (later to include social care) and it was clear to us that, although there was some positive involvement work occurring, this tended to happen in isolated pockets, with little sense in reality of there being a shared overarching vision outside of the SIG.

Early work focussed on attempting to establish exactly where existing involvement was happening, raising awareness in those areas where it was not and developing a better infrastructure for involvement, including an interim payments policy, information pack, involvement support group and newsletter. We initially held a stakeholder event to help inform this work.

Although the strategy itself was fairly non-prescriptive, one particular aim proved very useful to quote as a strategic aspiration, and this was that we should aim to 'culturally embed' involvement. In practice, it was hoped that this would translate into service users and carers being consistently involved in programmes, from inception to delivery and review.

Such activity did begin to grow, but it became apparent, as perhaps should have been expected, that one of the main challenges to culturally embedding involvement was to be the existing culture or, more accurately, different cultures within the School. Some branches of nursing, for example, have a more inclusive tradition within practice than others, so tended to be ahead of the game. In other disciplines it took time to conceptualise exactly how involvement might meaningfully occur or, indeed, whether it was relevant at all. In this regard we experienced some resistance to our understanding of involvement at an individual staff level, and difficulty in terms of traditional structures not always being conducive.

In tackling the first of these challenges, formal staff development opportunities were provided on an occasional basis in the early days, but these tended to attract the converted. Informal support has often proved much more productive. The degree to which academic colleagues would need personal support in taking forward the involvement agenda was largely unforeseen and still remains fairly unarticulated. They will not necessarily admit to feeling personally uncomfortable or unprepared for involvement work. For some it has been important that they receive support to start small and expand as their confidence improves.

Some of the structural challenges began to be tackled when, in 2007, steps were taken to disband the Strategy Implementation Group and initiate a new way of working. It was our view that the group had become marginal, in the grand scheme of things, and that the strategic responsibility for involvement in programmes should be 'owned' by the School Learning and Teaching Committee. In support of it taking on strategic direction, we set up an Involvement Advisory Group (IAG) made up of 50% service users/carers and 50% staff 'enthusiasts' (people with experience of doing involvement). The IAG now supports service user and carer involvement in learning, teaching and research across the School by meeting six times per year to come up with creative ideas for how involvement might take place and offer constructive suggestions to other staff seeking advice. Lunch is provided and discussion occurs in a friendly informal manner.

The working atmosphere fostered at the IAG is, we feel, much more conducive to this work than some of the more traditional committee-type structures that are common in universities. At a more fundamental level, we have recognised that respectful relationships are key to meaningful and sustained involvement. This has been a central feature of the service user and carer induction programme we have been running collaboratively with Faculty and other West Yorkshire university partners. Networking and collaborative working has been valuable in our endeavours because it has allowed us to lead, develop, draw on, and contribute to a strong national 'community of practice' for involvement; one which emphasises important values such as authenticity.

Emerging changes in how the School does business, particularly emphasizing a more integrated relationship between learning, teaching and research, means this is an opportune time for us to be looking closely at how involvement activity might change in response to current priorities, and the kind of infrastructure that might be needed to facilitate any strategic and methodological reframing in the future.

This work is just beginning, but we are keen to take forward the development of mutually beneficial knowledge transfer relationships, with health focussed community organisations, offering an opportunity for applying internal resources and sourced external community development/research funding to areas of work which could lead to substantive rewards for the School and the communities we engage with.

8.8   Final Words

The voices you have heard have been true reflections from the people involved in service user and carer involvement. They may resonate with you or be discordant to the voices you have heard. We would like to thank everyone for their contribution and hope you have found them thought provoking.

9 Making Sense of Involvement in Comensus

9.1 Introduction

At this juncture, we wish to turn to some qualitative research findings emerging from the Comensus project that illustrate the relevance of social movements theory in helping to make sense of service user and carer involvement in a university setting. Reflecting various foundational ideals and aspirations, the Comensus project is itself organised as a participatory action research study (Downe *et al.*, 2007, and elsewhere in this book). In this sense, the research element is co-constructed in an attempt to get away from a process of enquiry conducted on people, rather than produced collectively with them.

This book is itself one outcome of the work undertaken collectively under the Comensus banner. In one sense, this initiative can be viewed as an institutional response to policy supportive of increasing levels of public involvement in health and social care services, as this is acted out in health and social care education. Given the institutional nature of the initiative, there was (and continues to be) a risk of bureaucratic barriers to full empowerment and transformational change, and institutional tendencies towards co-option and incorporation. However, the underlying philosophy of the project aimed for the achievement of more aspirational outcomes (Marris and Rein, 1967; Marris, 1982). On a reflexive note, the staff involved in supporting the initiative reported personal commitments to more progressive principles of authentic alliances and long-standing relationships with certain health, welfare and disability movements (Downe *et al.*, 2007). Data collection within the action research cycles of the project has included asking explicit questions of participants including what led to their original involvement, and what sustains it.

In the various interviews and focus groups that have been run for the project, and in the records of routine meetings and events held as part of it, service user and carer participants' reflections are resonant with the sense that they are involved in some sort of social change. The talk is replete with motivations and aspirations to make a difference, and the processes by which this is to be achieved are essentially social in character, with relational aspects and interconnections between individuals and groups emphasised. Other elements focus on important issues of selfhood, identity and community. A selective presentation of some of these accounts illustrates some key connections between the talk of Comensus participants and the wider literature on social movements.

9.2 Making a Difference

Typically, starting with personal experiences as users of services or carers, participants'[1] accounts express a strong desire to make a difference. More often than not, these aspirations indicate the potential in some way to effect change in the actual delivery of health and social care services by influencing the development of future generations of practitioners, workforce training generally, or in the course of knowledge production by being involved in research:

> I tend to moan about things a lot but there is no point in just moaning. It is not just about being heard. It is more productive. You want to make a difference, to change things . . . (Brenda, interview)

> . . . the opportunity to bring out of ourselves something and offer it, . . . experiences, problems or whatever . . . If you can get in at the beginning you can make a vast difference. (Jacqui, interview)

The difference to be made can be quite specific, or hugely aspirational:

> The purpose of this group is to improve people's attitudes . . . about disability, mental health, learning difficulties. (John C, focus group)

> Amongst the CIT we have all had problems in dealing with health professionals. We are here to change things in the long term. (Robert, focus group)

> . . . great things: it could be an example for the way things are done all over the country . . . to get things right to have to involve people from the very beginning . . . (Kate)

Some participants locate their enthusiasm for change in a constructively critical stance:

> We are there to make a difference. It is not always about badgering on about negatives, though this sometimes has to happen. But it is about looking for positives all the time. (Brenda, interview)

Others know that the changes they seek may not be realised immediately, or could very well have been achieved previously with different circumstances:

> Keep chipping away: it might take a long time but you get there eventually. (John C, focus group)

> . . . this should have occurred years ago. (Lillian)

---

[1] The term 'participant' is used here to denote the various service users and carers involved in this participatory action research project. It may have been preferable to use a more collegiate term such as 'colleague' to reflect the sense of joint enterprise between academic staff, service users and carers, but this may also have been confusing for readers.

Concern with the idea of pace of change was not just an issue in terms of achieving transformational objectives in the work of the university or health and social care services. It was also important in relation to the internal organization of Comensus, emerging structures and processes of decision making.

For example, an early decision to develop organizational approaches at a steady and accessible pace, so as not to exclude those with less experience of meetings and organizing, those with particular impairments, or those initially short on confidence, created some tension with those who wanted to press on quickly:

> Pace frustrating but essential – Moving from planning and organisation to involvement and action. (Nat)

Reflections on the process of decision making on the part of one Community Involvement Team (CIT) member are resonant with some of the observations on a prefigurative standpoint (Chapter 2):

> Better decisions are taken, including the decision about how long to deliberate. (John L)

> Problems with social decision making: (the need to) reduce to a minimum the maximum amount of distress caused. (John L)

Another participant articulates how her long-term ambitions for involvement have developed. Through linking these to a rejection of certain organizational formalities, she arrives at a more radical perspective:

> ... at one point I had stated that I felt we should concentrate on our experience rather than trying to change the world . . . . In fact, I do think we should be changing the world, and I think that this project can definitely do that. [it] was the approach: one contributor seemed to be fixated on looking at many other committees and organisations and trying to work out who is doing what and reorganizing them all, but I felt that we would get bogged down with this approach (as this person seemed to be) and that our starting point had to be our own valuable and very relevant experiences. From that starting point we can go on to change the world, but it has to be very much grass roots up, and not the other way around. (Kate, written feedback)

The extent to which participants in a university involvement initiative can exert influence on health and social care practice and services is constrained by the indirect nature of the activity. The input is targeted on the next generation of practitioners and managers, or the continuing education of the current workforce. Project participants commented on this in the context of the relative ease with which a change agenda might be taken up in different settings:

> ... The culture [in services] does not allow people like myself to have a very strong voice ... and it felt like a constant battle, fighting for what we needed ... [in Comensus] ... more service users or carers led than anything I have seen before. (Kate)

> short cut into the system by being inside the university. (Paul, focus group)

> Getting in at the beginning. Learning is one thing, relating to a person is another thing. (Jacqui)

> ... closed doors before unless you wanted to be re-educated by the university. This is different: we are re-educating them. (Les, focus group)

A strong vein of altruism runs through many of the aspirations for change and personal motivations to take part in the project in the first place and persists with continuing involvement:

you do your own bit so that everyone benefits. I might not personally benefit from it in my lifetime ... I realised I had taken things out of society all my life, and now I can put something back. (John C, focus group)

I would like the teachers to get out of it what I get out of it. I would like them to get some sense of, not just fulfilment, a deeper change at the personal level. It should be a meaningful experience for them as a person. Not just practical changes, but of course, that as well. (Brenda, interview)

Can see the potential to improve the plight of people with dyspraxia by influencing health professionals and promoting change. ... I am constantly fighting not just for myself but trying to change things for other people having similar predicaments. (Robert, focus group)

My experience after I lost my leg was that after being discharged from hospital I was completely on my own, no counselling, no follow-up. My only form of transport was the wheelchair. Could not get around at all because of the lack of drop kerbs, narrow doorways and so on. Public transport, same sort of problems. I hope I can help solve some of these problems so people can benefit from it. (John C, focus group)

This concern for the welfare of others can be linked to personal empowerment and confidence building:

how a person makes their own voice...and can help the other people ... (Nat, focus group)

It can also be linked to recognition of common humanity and everyone's potential to be a service user at some time in their lives:

Each of us occupies each other's position at some stage in the past, or the future, and we are interested in making [this] as good as it can possibly be (John L, interview)

Some are motivated and sustained in their involvement by powerful emotions and are passionate about their involvement:

I am still like that [angry]. I get frustrated with policy makers and bureaucrats. I am constantly gritting my teeth with the incompetence of policy and the lack of thought and insight into people's needs ... I can turn this anger into something positive by fighting back, not giving up. (Robert, focus group)

[When first disabled] Felt like giving up, everything was against me, demoralised. Had to get hold of myself – "are you going to give in, or are you going to fight?" Decided to act and join the access group. (John C, focus group)

This can connect with other emotions which arise from participation:

Pride in Comensus, and in what we have achieved, because it is effective. I remember ... being really angry about how I might be perceived ... Wanted to have a say about people's language and attitudes especially as it relates to ethnicity. (Brenda, interview)

9.3   Collective Identity

Despite the diverse backgrounds and experiences of the Community Involvement Team as a whole, individuals quickly divined common identity in the use of health and social care services or caring roles. Lived experiences, personal attributes and talents, are fore-grounded in these user or carer narratives and are collectively valued:

> We bring all the expertise together in one go. (Robert, focus group)

> .... Although disabled, a lot to offer ... We have talents over and above ... Comensus allows us to use all our skills. (Nat)

Much of the teaching and learning that takes place with service user and carer input draws heavily on the personal experiences and biographies of respective participants. People tell their stories in an attempt to advance student learning or share snapshots of personal experience to emphasise particular points. In the university, this sort of thing can take place in the course of meetings with staff or peers, as well as in the classroom. When this goes well, there is often a positive reciprocation of respect, appreciation, or empathy for people's experiences and perhaps even some collective discussion that may assist in making sense of it. This willingness for students to engage authentically with service users and carers can add to the experience of being personally valued for those doing the presentation.

In the course of engagement in an initiative like Comensus, all those involved become increasingly aware of each others' personal stories, talents and strengths, the detail of which may have been relatively hidden to start with. A number of members of the Community Involvement Team ended up taking responsibility for quite specific pieces of work because they possessed specific relevant skills. For example, one member who was quite shy at first, turned out to be an accomplished graphic artist and went on to design a logo for the group. Increasing knowledge of the range of different strengths in the group and people's unique biographies has assisted in the distribution of work. This has created a complementary linking together of different people's expertise and mutual support within the group, approximating somewhat to the Marxist aphorism of 'from each according to their ability, to each according to their need'. These emergent phenomena also strongly reinforce the argument of Freire, that education can be mutually empowering for teacher and student where there is authentic desire for learning that is not constrained by institutional norms and boundaries.

This approach also generates a sense of solidarity and mutual support that engenders feelings of safety in expressing views and feelings. This is typically mentioned in terms of feeling valued in the context of working together and how this translates into feelings of belonging. This is contrasted with prior experiences of being devalued and can be associated with the previously mentioned altruism:

Disability can make you a non person, project gives belonging ... Really I did not feel anyone valued anything I said or did until I joined the access group or started doing disability awareness training ... Here we are looked at in terms of what we can do, not what we cannot do ... A sense of value comes in when you know you can help somebody. (John C, focus group)

A more positive view of self was linked to giving and getting respect within the Community Involvement Team and in interaction with university staff and students:

because their minds have opened as to how they can help. (Hasumati)

they listened and I think they were keen to listen. (Phil)

Or linked to overcoming personal crises:

Being accepted and coming to meetings helped me through. (John L, focus group)

This sense of being valued is reciprocated and reflected in other relationships, enabling people to be themselves:

Comensus values rather than devalues ... not only does the university value, but so do we – we value the university, our other partners, and the others we meet. (Les, focus group)

Seeing how others have done, motivates me. (Phil, focus group)

[It] goes beyond self advocacy in engaging with teaching and research.
      I feel that because I know that I belong my views are accepted, accepted just for me, I do not feel personally that I have to modify my behaviour. In other places I have to shape my behaviour. (CIT Brenda, interview)

Notwithstanding the evident diversity within the group, the overarching feeling is of shared experience and occupying common ground:

When you have got something in common with someone it kind of creates a space where you can off-load ... say I want to talk about [issue] find it easier to raise issues with people like me, with shared experiences. Feel safe and comfortable to say things. ... When you have got something in common with someone it kind of creates a space where you can offload ... and feeling comfortable to raise issues. In a different way using maybe different language than with say professionals. (Brenda, focus group)

For this participant there is also a sense of how this identity is shaped and evolves in the course of group activities:

The fact that we are in Comensus sometimes shapes the way that we think and what we do. The groups that you are in ... you are learning, sharing knowledge about what your group is about, what it is ... helps move forward. (Brenda, focus group)

Though the participants seldom refer to themselves in the language of activism, it is easy to see them as activists for the user movement and their local communities. Some views resonate with wider protest movements:

Today, people say, global warming, save the world, and I agree with that. But on disability issues you have got to start local. So many things need changing . . . We have all got things in common. They have got a goal, a reason, a meaning in life. They are getting on and doing something about it. (John C, focus group)

There is an appreciation of collective strength and solidarity.

after the first couple of [Comensus] meetings you recognised the people you have got there have everything covered. All disabilities, it is a very powerful position. (John C, focus group)

developed a sense of solidarity and familiarity . . . settled into the environment [university] . . . We get together as a group, we get to know each other, we have a similar cause, we share experience. This is solidarity. (Robert, focus group)

This reflects an ethos of team working:

[Previously] Biggest part of [my] life was being self employed. A big problem to start with was not having what I said being done. But now really appreciate being part of a team. You feel stronger working as a group than working individually. Confidence comes out of group strength. (John C, focus group)

Action is grounded in experience and potential strength is articulated in terms that link the collective with the personal:

Service users and carers share experiences of suffering and adversity . . . We have had to battle and fight to get our rights. When I was younger my parents were fobbed off by professionals. Now I have developed assertiveness, ability to fight corner politically and engage in action. Now I will not accept no for an answer. (Robert, focus group)

Things are beginning to come together and helping me to feel better about myself and stronger about myself. I have been asked to do things that are important to other organisations. (Paul, focus group)

9.4 Relationships

There is a significant emphasis on relationships amongst Community Involvement Team members. These relational aspects and personal connections are the basis for cooperation, support and enthusiasm within the group. Occasionally, individuals experience a worsening of their health conditions, or other life stresses, which invariably elicit support and assistance from other group members:

you notice about people's individual problems and you work together on it, offer support. (John C, focus group)

Not everyone begins with the same level of confidence, but group cohesion soon develops:

At first it took me a bit to get into it, but I have enjoyed getting involved. Initially I was insecure, because of the newness of the situation, new people, new ideas. Did not know too much what you were walking into. (Robert, focus group)

The quality of interpersonal connections can move beyond merely establishing effective working relationships, and can develop into friendships:

> Through the project I have made new friends and gained new contacts. Find it beneficial to share experiences with people ... especially when people listen. (Robert, focus group)

> I can get to know other people and get things changed (Phil, focus group)

> friendship ... we all get along. In other groups it is all work ... we get things done in an easier way (Paul, focus group)

These relationships are sustained in the course of activities focused on group objectives but the group also meets socially and recreationally, further strengthening friendly relations.

9.5   Linking to Wider Networks

Membership of, and connections to, established groups and networks (both self-organised user and carer groups and more broadly based community groups) greatly assisted in initially recruiting people to Comensus:

> recruiting people was not just ... an advert ... encouragement from people outside of the project who saw the publicity material and pointed it out to people they thought might be good candidates (Hasumati, focus group)

> I have always been in protests as part of groups ... Protests about disability access issues for instance. ... Would not have known about it [Comensus] without that group. ... Joined Comensus through DISC. They introduced me to it. (John C, focus group)

Participants bring perspectives and experiences forged in different groups and communities as part of their contribution to Comensus:

> I think the personal thing is really important because sometimes people might not have contact with black people. Their only knowledge is not directly from black people themselves ... I am able to make sure those things are visible within our project (Brenda, interview)

Membership of the Community Involvement Team enables some participants to discover new connections, opening up membership to other groups they were previously unaware of:

> [named member] and me joined Preston mental heath service user forum. (Robert, focus group)

For others, these connections helped facilitate extensions of support between different groups, including the promotion of mutual appreciation for each other's issues and causes:

> I was on the Caribbean Women's Forum and also volunteer with Sure Start ... I helped another CIT member to do some diabetes research. I helped her group to better design

their questionnaire and make introductions into the African and Caribbean community. (Brenda, interview)

Similarly, membership of the Community Involvement Team enables individuals to appreciate and support each other's issues and causes:

For me, in Sure Start, if a grandma comes in I might talk a lot more because I have picked up on issues for older people. (Brenda, interview)

9.6 Positive Effects of Involvement

Despite many people coming to the group with an explicit agenda to help others, after time they reported various positive effects for themselves. These benefits include developing confidence and assertiveness and a range of practical skills. They are clearly linked to action in the minds of the participants:

People are moving forward in their lives by helping other people. (Hasumati, focus group)

Through getting people involved they get confidence. . . . Things you have fought hard for and eventually get it, you appreciate it more. (John C, focus group)

9.7 Discussion

Touraine's (1978) concept of 'historicity' – linking capacity for self-reflective and creative social action with social struggles – is mirrored in many of the accounts. Similarly, Touraine's theorizing on the futility of predicting the direction and form that social change might take is relevant to the acknowledgement from within the Community Involvement Team that institutional practices cannot be transformed immediately. Expressed aspirations for change also concede that the group works towards an unknown and unknowable future. Comensus members seek access to information and knowledge which will assist themselves and generations to come.

There are clear connections with Melucci's concerns with the development of a collective identity grounded in everyday interaction, rather than one which is imposed and the strongly linked view of movements as sponsors of meaning. The annual 'One In Four' film festival (at the Mitchell and Kenyon Cinema, University of Central Lancashire), a user-led initiative aimed at tackling stigma around mental health, exemplifies the way in which university staff and students can come together with the community to promote change and understanding. Typically, the screening of a film is followed by an open discussion of relevant issues, often facilitated by someone who has personal experiences that connect with these cinematic representations. Tutors can bring what they learn from such initiatives into the classroom, the lecture hall and into public, organised debates, offering the university a more active role in its community, and citizens a more active role in the life of the university. A key element of all of this is a contribution to the process by which stigmatised identity is reflected upon, faced up to, and rejected.

The importance of relationships within the group is stressed by Community Involvement Team members, mirroring Castells' (1996) theory that meaning is produced in the bringing into being of a movement, regardless of its achievements. This centrality of relational issues and shared experience highlights a convergence of public and private spheres and supports Offe's (1987) account of movements fashioning their own space from where to raise questions.

Other comments indicating awareness of wider protest movements and participants' links with other community groups and networks support Castells' (1996) view that the production of meaning is not limited to activists, but broadens out to the wider community. Resistance to powerful ideologies, particularly medical hegemony, can also be found, which is recognizably important as a first step for enacting social change. Linked to this is some evidence of shared socio-political values (Offe, 1985, 1987; Rothschild-Whitt, 1979) and a powerful sense of 'what could be'.

Delanty's (2003) construct of personalism as an alternative form of individualism is reflected in the accounts of what motivated people to become involved, and how their enthusiasm and commitment are sustained. In this regard, altruistic motives and aspirations for change are prominent in contradiction of rational-choice analyses. These impulses can also be discerned in some of the reflections on team working and collective identity. Such factors also exemplify the notion of intrinsic movement goals identified by Klandermans (1997). There is evidence that indignation and anger at experiences in health and social care services feeds a sense of injustice that, in turn, adds to people's motivation to make a difference. This linking of emotions to collective action in social movements has been highlighted in numerous other contexts (Barker, 2001).

Rothschild-Whitt's (1979) ideal type of organization within social movements shares many features with the experiences in the Comensus project. The Community Involvement Team members have developed their own organizational structures and process, which are non-hierarchical and egalitarian, involve consensual decision making and a strong sense of solidarity and community. This, and the value placed upon relational aspects of organization, is evocative of the notion of prefiguration that is associated with many social movements. The everyday kindnesses and mutual support transacted in the act of organizing for involvement echo the feminist inspired prominence of relationships in establishing a trade union at Harvard University (Hoerr, 1997). The attempts to structure decision making and meetings to suit the needs of participants and avoid hierarchy draws a parallel with a long tradition of Utopian and affinity-based principles (Day, 2005). The nature of reported interactions, the qualities that individuals bring to them, and their emotional as well as practical dimensions, offer a prefiguration of better social relations within the university for the benefit of all, including students and academic staff.

The motivations espoused by many of the Comensus members emphasise altruistic hopes for others and the desire to make a difference. This supports

Rothschild-Whitt's (1979) taxonomy of incentives, with common purpose being the main reason for getting and staying involved. Arguably, this raises the potential for resilience in the face of institutional pulls toward bureaucratization and co-option.

The theoretical and reflective literature on social movements and social change discussed in Chapter 2 connects with the service user and carer narratives presented here at a number of levels. In this chapter, quotes have been selected from Community Involvement Team members that illustrated these sort of connections to make the point that it is important to realise that service user and carer involvement initiatives do share features of organisation and experience with broader movements for social change. However, as noted in Chapter 2, this does not mean that university involvement *is* a social movement. Rather, the journey of finding out and making sense of involvement can be informed by recourse to movement knowledge and theory, and this may in turn improve participants' chances of realising their personal and collective goals to make a difference and resist forces of co-option and incorporation. Similarly, academic staff who relate to involvement participants and their associated groups can become more aware of these movement dimensions and begin to consider their own behaviour and support in this light. This may mean simply making more of an effort to strive for authenticity rather than instrumentality in these relationships. Or, more interestingly, there may be a raised potential for building alliances that bridge service user and professional interests.

10 Shedding Masks: Transitions in Mental Health and Education, a Personal View

William Park

Don't think Disability, think ABILITY.

10.1 Introduction

Individuals who succeed in managing and overcoming mental health 'conditions' can go on to provide *insights* for others. Supportive groups and service user involvement in higher education have their valuable place, but individuals, ultimately, need to rise to their life's potential, and be in a position to inspire.

My standpoint in this short chapter is one of sympathy and shared purpose when it comes to service user groups. I have had meaningful links with three such groups in Preston. But the key to progress for me has been a range of activities and coping strategies, an inner sense of purpose, followed by a move back to a career path (tutoring) which links to my previous experience in writing and adult education tutoring. This is a path forged from *within*.

I am concerned that everyone maintains a sense of moving forward. Eventually, for many, that will mean a transition *beyond* the role, term and label that is 'service user'. I believe the key lies in education. Those involved in the educational process have a responsibility to enhance people's full potential.

10.2 Rejecting the Label of Service User

The term 'service user' has a poor status, in my view. Imagine the scene – a conference filled with professors, lecturers, and so on, but at 'question time' one introduces oneself as a 'service user'. I have been at some excellent conferences, but I refuse to introduce myself in this way anymore. I would go so far as to say, it is demeaning. The term limits and defines one negatively. This is partly due to status and issues of hierarchy. If one introduces oneself as a healthcare professional, one immediately possesses a higher status. Attached to that status is income and power. Conferences are filled with highly-paid professionals.

I know the Comensus initiative at the University of Central Lancashire (UCLan) does its best to remunerate contributions from service users, but, welcome though this is, they are token amounts, and, quite simply, however much service users enjoy greater participation in the life of the university, the fact is they are surrounded by well-paid professionals and administrators and so the hierarchical structure remains. It is reinforced every single day by the appellation 'service user'. Many service users I have spoken to dislike this label, so how did it come about, and why does it remain? I do not hear anyone calling themselves a 'service provider', even if they are one.

Service user involvement in higher education is a *stage* along the way, not a lifestyle choice. There is a danger in successful 'service user' groups being marginalised as curiosities, tamed by the structures supporting them, and not actually impacting directly on changing attitudes in the wider world – I mean the man and woman on the street. It is clear that where service user groups have been successful is in raising the esteem of the participants, as well as gently and cumulatively altering the 'attitudes' of healthcare professionals, and reinforcing the already enlightened attitudes of interested specialist health groups working in the community.

One should not be 'ashamed' of one's 'condition' but should one be 'proud' either? I have outlined my concerns over terminology and power structures. Freedom involves freedom from restrictive labels, true opportunities for remunerative involvement, community engagement, and an emphasis on people going beyond one's unhappiest state and being autonomous as *individuals*, not simply as members of various collaborative groups. University initiatives like Comensus, emphasizing service user involvement, are laudable in intention and promote self-esteem for the service user participants, but I believe, given perceptions of the wider general public outside of university establishments, that much needs to be done in the community at large to promote education around mental health issues.

Service users repeatedly talking about their illnesses, or 'conditions', is a reminder to themselves of their illnesses, and reinforces the prism of that identity...the minute they are well or better again, they may still be identified as a 'survivor' or 'ex' service user...one survives, like a victim of personal devastation...as though whatever 'condition' one had originally, is always potentially in danger of returning. I believe, if attitudes and perceptions changed, individuals could reach a plateau where 'illness' could be seen as a construct left behind long ago, never to return. In fact, it could be argued that disability itself is a social, political and economic creation.

As things stand, 'service users' have a great willingness to participate in projects and discussions; meanwhile, in political, social and economic terms they are often marginalised as dysfunctional. This has to change, and I believe the way forward is in collaborative education of the kind espoused by Paulo Freire (1971). I will return to Freire a little later, but his approach underpins my thinking throughout this chapter.

10.3   Involvement and Self-actualization

True opportunity and advancement is in the world of *mainstream* work and society, where people pay taxes, experience loss, rewards, disappointments and happiness, and where people encounter others of greater or lesser sophistication than themselves. It is this world that, I would hope, the 'service user' is guided towards, with assistance from education. But if the machinery of education in institutions is founded on 'delivering' information, merely ticking the boxes for a range of 'delivered' systems, which managers can then be 'proud' of, then true advancement is compromised from the beginning.

For service users or carers, there need be no contradiction in actualizing the self and being generous and humane to others. This extends to the content of contributions to teaching and scholarly activity. People who have overcome particular life problems could emphasise the creativity and individualisation they have used to overcome difficulties, rather than the difficulties themselves. This in itself can be a political act, or form of praxis. In the context of mental health, for example, it can extend to efforts to combat the climate of fear generated by the media (the mentally ill as useless, troubled or downright dangerous) with more considered, humanitarian approaches, in tune with contemporary interest in the principal of recovery but resisting conservative forces which would dilute its radical potential (Pilgrim, 2008).

Education surely values intelligence and insight, but these are not necessarily dependent on advanced literary or intellectual gifts. Rather, they can be grounded in the experience of a range of tutors and teachers sensitive and brave enough to inspire and encourage. For lay teachers, a productive way these can be achieved is by accessing personal resources of courage and self-belief, even in the face of individual health difficulties, such as mental 'deterioration'. It may well be that it is the damaged sensitives, the creative rebels, the burnt-out intellectual radicals who prove to have the most powerful and pertinent arguments.

What is clear to me is that most people are involved in a distraction from the responsibility towards realizing their own potential. This is the tragedy for every single human, whether it be the pressure to conform, the pressures of family, the lack of material wealth, or the inadequate help individuals may get when confronted with perhaps the most dynamic and important phase of their lives – a period of mental ill health. I believe, too, that *medication* is simply a stage along the way towards better health for those with mental health problems, and needs to be seen in a context of other helping factors; including personal creativity, resilience and resourcefulness.

Diversions and pressures to succeed in conventional terms (money, property and family life) take up most of people's time, generally, and force us into role-playing at home and work. The kind of success and achievement I am espousing is based on an *inner* personal journey, whether this is spiritual, creative or simply being 'true' to oneself.

This is not something that can be *given* by others, however well-meaning, or, as Freire (1971: 39) explained it: via 'an egoism cloaked in the false generosity of paternalism'.

In the epigraph to Will Self's novel *Dorian: An Imitation* (2002), Schopenhauer is quoted as saying:

> There is an unconscious appositeness in the use of the word person to designate the human individual, as is done in all European languages: for persona really means an actor's mask, and it is true that no one reveals himself as he is; we all wear a mask and play a role.

For some, the mask fragments and slips entirely. They may then be labelled with terms that, unfortunately, set them apart: manic-depressive, schizophrenic, depressed, neurotic or personality-disordered. Furthermore, if they seek help, they are then lumbered with another limiting label: 'service user'. I have come to the conclusion that I am none of these. This rejection of externally imposed labels connects with commentary in Chapter 2 regarding the features of health and welfare social movements.

10.4 My Self, a Personal View

If pressed, I will say now I have bouts of CSA – a term I have originated, standing for Creative Suicidal Anxiety. CSA means being over-sensitive, with a leaning towards imaginative/creative expression, possibly in the arts. The sufferer often senses a dichotomy between the inner world of the imagination and the social, practical reality. This can produce a feeling of sometimes panicky or destructive over-anxiety, inwardness, and not wanting to face the world. Such sensitivity can lead to times of intense thinking, but this can be draining too, with periods of lethargy. There is also an increased sensitivity to noise. However, this sensitivity, also apparent towards people in regard to sensing other people's feelings, can potentially be a positive quality. The trouble is that the hyper-awareness can be chaotic and sometimes overwhelming. It needs to be harnessed. I have recognised the need to channel the awareness creatively, along with calming the mind periodically. Now I focus using meditation; in the past, I used to dampen my over-active mind with alcohol.

My need for perfection, to embrace everything philosophically so to speak, is often difficult to manage, and some of my 'attempts' can lead to reams of notes, ideas spiralling and connecting, words highlighted with coloured pens. It can be difficult to abandon objects too, as their relative significance or insignificance can be in doubt. Sometimes there is crippling reactive depression due to remorse and regret, when relationships have been affected. I call all of this 'CSA'. It is certainly not 'straightforward' depression!

But, whether I have 'CSA' stamped on my psyche, or not, what I do know is that I have been involved with various mental health 'service user' groups over the past year, one based in a university (UCLan), and now I have had a range and variety of help from the 'services' too, I feel I can make progress with my background in adult education tutoring. With a part-time plan, and eventually a full-time post, I hope, I aim to develop my tutoring interests in creative writing, adult literacy, meditation and well-being, and film studies – I am something of a cineaste, though have no formal qualification in this area.

The annual 'One In Four' film festival[1], as well as the excellent *Barbershop* magazine[2], are indicative of projects that can promote change and understanding. Tutors can bring what they learn from such initiatives into the classroom, the lecture hall and into public, organised debates. Of the latter, arguably, there should be many more, specifically for the general public – to combat ignorance and stigma.

10.5   Redemptive Education

What is important, in experiencing an illness, or educating others, is *conveying humanity*, so that we, and others *together*, can understand at the deepest level and go further, and achieve more, perhaps, than those who are presently teaching us. The medical establishment, and its maladaptive responses to mental ill health, needs to be supplemented by enlightened approaches in the education sector, and in the creative arts, and these to be combined with individual initiatives. The purpose of further and higher education is surely to activate our best, highest selves? For those who are conventionally 'well' and those who have suffered periods of instability: a reaching towards intellectual, artistic and spiritual success.

Abraham Maslow (1994: 180, 183) in *The Farther Reaches of Human Nature* says 'one of the goals of education should be to teach that life is precious' and 'another goal of education is to refreshen the consciousness so that we are continually aware of the beauty and wonder of life'. Maslow speaks of how 'unlike the current model of teacher as lecturer, conditioner, reinforcer and boss, the Taoist helper or teacher is *receptive* rather than intrusive' (Maslow, 1994: 181, author's emphasis). In this context, Taoistic is 'asking rather than telling. It means non-intruding, non-controlling. It stresses non-interfering observation rather than a controlling manipulation. It is receptive and passive rather than active and forceful' (Maslow, 1994: 14).

Maslow's recommendation for a facilitative, receptive teaching style reflects a strand of humanism, of informed compassion allied to wisdom that has been significant in shaping progressive models of adult education and participatory approaches to development and research. Freire (1971: 29), in his seminal book

---

[1] User-led Film Festival that takes place annually in the Mitchell and Kenyon Cinema, UCLan: www.uclan.ac.uk/health/news/film_festival.php.

[2] Produced by the mental health race equality team, Central Lancashire Primary Care Trust: www.centrallancashire.nhs.uk/DocImages/406.pdf.

Pedagogy of the Oppressed, talks about how emancipation needs to be an 'act of love' and people's education and advancement are not prescribed, but learning and understanding is a mutual collaborative effort. With his emphasis on relational aspects of learning and liberation it is not surprising that Freire has informed the thinking of movement scholars and activists interested in prefigurative ideals (Chapter 2). These ideas have been thoroughly taken up in progressive developments in education and research, such as action learning and action research (Chapter 4).

There is a need for 'reflection' says Freire, followed by 'action' (1971: 38). The attitude of oppressors can be inherently demeaning to the underprivileged, confusing material disadvantage with incompetence or laziness, missing completely the potential in every human being. Freire was initially concerned with the poor and illiterate in Brazil, but his theories of learning, social change and compassion for the underdog could just as well be applied to those stigmatised and excluded on grounds of disability or health condition. Highlighting action for change, Freire is keen to point out that a conviction for the right to freedom (of thought, of opportunity) 'cannot be packaged and sold' (Freire 1971: 54). In other words, for the disadvantaged, those in need, the oppressed, the urge for freedom and authentic advancement must come *from within*. As Freire (1971: 55) says, management, also, is an 'arm' of domination and cannot be the instrument for securing people's rights and potential for growth.

Freire's egalitarian social ideals are matched in his view of the proper relationship between teacher and student. The 'revolutionary educator . . . must be a partner of the students in his relations with them' (Freire 1971: 62). This admits of a concept, similar to karmic interaction, whereby people are not passive and separate from the world and each other, but are rather *active* and mutually *acting* participants. The role of education and the educator eschews the simple delivery of 'subject matter' for exploration and facilitation of all of the participants' resourcefulness and capacity for mutual support and collaboration. This would include engaging with people's inner sensitivity, awareness and mental potential, so that true learning as an aspect of *freedom* is experienced. Most importantly, this requires the educator/tutor to be prepared for an inner journey of their own, where they too are learning and adapting to the needs of others. Within these relationships, mutual respect is fostered between educator and educated, where roles interchange, based on common humanity, not grounded in status. Any prospective 'tutor' who has faith in their own inner being, and the inner self of others, is bound to elicit respect, and be a source of hope and leadership. It follows that an essential quality of such a Freirian educator is not just a sure grasp of their subject, but a capacity for completely honest self-reflection.

10.6 Alliances in Action

The potential for alliances between university staff and service users can take interesting courses in the context of a university, especially if there is a commitment from within to become a critically engaged institution in relation to the local community (Chapter 3). If individuals have the bravery and wisdom of an independent approach, free from ideological or bureaucratic tendencies to institutional reaction, progress can happen. Educators, lay and professional tutors amongst them, can then give of themselves as unique, honest individuals, prepared to speak their mind and to have an impact in the wider community (for instance, in public speaking or in public seminars). They need courage to speak from the heart, and not just to be a spokesperson for an institution. Moreover, greater community engagement can begin to mobilise the resources of the university, for community benefit. For projects and activities involving 'service users', there should be real equality, not hierarchy. This permits an organic learning process for all, where the value of each individual is recognised and the resultant 'community' prefigures the society we would aspire to achieve.

For Freire (1971: 130), 'dialogue is the essence of revolutionary action' and without doubt dialogue and discussion has underpinned the progress of Comensus. The latter point reinforces Freire's (1971: 114) views on the importance of using the 'best channel of communication'. In this respect the Comensus initiative has been enlightened, utilising a varied use of videos and presentations and, within their published output and minutes of meetings, for example, a clarifying employment of symbols and language.

This dialogic stance, however, needs to be continuously revived and maintained through the individual qualities of the participants. It is not something that can be prescribed, nor is it wholly free from the more covert threats implicit in impenetrable academic or medical terminology and imbalances of power. Arguably, universities are caught between egalitarian impulses and conservative reaction en route to both increasing participation and also consolidating insularity and elitism. The latter elements comprise the sort of prescribed ways of doing and thinking that, for Freire (1971: 153), includes a precept 'not to think'. This echoes Chomsky's remark that 'education is a system of imposed ignorance'[3]. The transformation of such systems offers routes to re-ordering patterns of status and esteem, and renegotiation of identities for participants, both service users and academic staff.

For the academics involved, renouncing patterns of domination, however subtle or possibly well meaning in origin, can be problematic and include 'a threat to their own identities' (Freire, 1971: 154). It is so important, then, that honest discussion and the opportunity and time for this, forms a part of collective relationships. This Freirian manifesto involves 'an act of love and true commitment' (Freire, 1971:162) and cannot be achieved by participants hiding behind masks or established roles, fearfully holding on to a sense of order, control and safety. Freire (1971: 183) warns us that a feeling of being 'hopeless and fearful of risking experimentation' leads to a condition whereby 'true creativity' is impossible.

---

[3] Taken from the documentary film *Manufacturing Comsent: Noam Chomsky and the Media*, directed by Mark Achbar and Peter Wintonick, 1992.

10.7 Conclusions

In conclusion, severe mental disturbance or mastery of a peaceful mind are both aspects of being human, but they are also an indicator of difference from the norm. We all want to feel safe and part of a crowd, but sometimes differences can take us forward. Potentials lie within us . . .let us by all means help each other, but give ourselves the freedom and the right to concentrate on healing our own weaknesses and developing our own strategies – this is self-education.

The best way to combat stigma about mental illness is to set a good example, fighting and overcoming one's own problems, and then exploring one's own creative, intellectual or spiritual capacities. Arguably, one role of educators and service user groups is to promote this. The gift of igniting people's own inner resources is the challenge for educators, a matter of guidance, inspiration and wisdom, not political or bureaucratic advancement. It involves the gift of being human, with all one's vulnerability, honesty and generosity.

Conclusions

The Importance and Value of Service User and Carer Involvement

Within this book, we have extensively discussed key issues in service user and carer involvement and examined real-world practical examples. You will have seen from Chapter 1 that there is a plethora of critical literature focusing on involvement, describing initiatives and making recommendations for good practice. That chapter also identified barriers to involvement and examined various ladders and continuums of involvement that have been developed to enable the evaluation of initiatives and hence ensure involvement is truly authentic.

Chapter 2 put this work in context, debated wider socio-political factors and examined theories of community and social movements. Radical change may very well be realizable within university systems of involvement, and this may have features similar to those found in social movements. Such analyses need to be tempered by the acknowledgement that incorporation and co-option tendencies also exist. Arguably, transformative change can be best achieved through progressive alliances between service users/carers and staff. We arrive at this conclusion from a perspective taken within such an alliance closely integrated to the university. It may well be that the most radical transformative goals are more likely to be actioned by groups independent of the university. Regardless of whether involvement initiatives are considered in terms of movement theory, the potential to bring about various changes is real. These might include a levelling of power relationships and initiation of new or shared identities that challenge notions of constructed difference and foreground our common humanity.

The examination of community engagement and progressive features of social enterprise within Chapter 3 identified how fulfilling and rewarding relationships can be catalysed by partnership working between academics, local communities and individual service users and carers. Mutual support and quality of relationships were seen to be central and valued features of successful involvement within universities, and prefigurative relational forms of organization that harnessed individual and collective creativity and agency emerge on route to the achievement of goals.

Chapter 4 focused on methods and outcomes that might be relevant for evaluation of such health and social care practitioner education programmes. The chapter drew on international literature, with some specific examples of service user/carer involvement in the context of the United States.

Taking the subject of evaluation and outcomes measurement further, Chapter 5 reviewed the contested nature of success and considered how difficult it may be to measure. It identified the range of potential stakeholders in the engagement enterprise, and the potential tensions between success for market-driven universities, and for individual service user and carer contributors. The theoretical purpose of higher education for health and social care staff was examined, alongside concepts of expertise and emotional intelligence, and of salutogenic as opposed to pathogenic outcome measures. The chapter proposed that the narrative structure that characterises service user and carer encounters in universities was ideally suited to an examination of the complex emergent nature of health and social care.

In Chapter 6 we examined the practicalities and journey of a real-life project – Comensus. The review covered a five-year period, investigating processes and activities. From this examination barriers and solutions to involvement were identified. The chapter explored the concept of culture within an academic setting and how this impacts on the initiative. It concluded with the message that enduring cultural change could only occur if all parties were authentically attached to altruistic and equity-based values that truly defined a service user/carer led initiative.

Chapter 7 took a different perspective, that of a manager, whose role was to support the growth of service user and carer involvement within the organization. It pointed out that strategic influence and the power to make change were key factors for successful project implementation. The author highlighted that resources are a major consideration for integrating and supporting involvement and, finally, concludes that this process of inclusion was continuous and one for which to strive constantly.

The next chapter comprised stories of engagement – personal accounts of involvement from a variety of authors. It covered key issues, lessons learnt and personal experiences. All the contributors to this section espoused their belief in the value of service user and carer involvement. Many reported positive benefits and effects. These experiences, however, were varied, not homogeneous. They also reflected some of the struggles and tensions in relationships with university systems and personnel and with each other. It is important that we also consider these difficulties and differences in making sense of the involvement experience and affording insights into the pursuit of lasting change.

Chapter 9 returns to some of the themes and theories presented in Chapter 2, demonstrating connections between these and reflection on the recorded talk of participants in the Comensus action research study.

Chapter 10 was a personal piece reflecting on selfhood and looking beyond the label of service user. The author believes that educators have a part in igniting people's inner resources, so that they can then explore their creative, intellectual and spiritual capacities. Hence, activities should not simply focus on internal organizational drivers for involvement.

Authenticity and Action

Service user and carer involvement is, for us, about valuing people's experiences. These are unique to individuals who have been service users or carers (rather than staff, teachers or researchers). The aim is to better inform teaching and research in health and related practice. This works at a number of different levels. In one sense this could be just about all the practicalities of organizing people to contribute to the various different forms of academic work (teaching, research, planning, evaluation etc.) from a personal perspective (i.e. informed by experience of service use or a caring role). Success could be measured in terms of volume and quality of the range of contributions. We would call this an 'instrumental' understanding of the involvement. In our view there is more than this at stake; the personal becomes the political.

People tell us their involvement is about effecting change, primarily in the university, but ultimately in the world of practice. In this sense, the involvement is a 'transformative' activity. Some of the change is material, working on systems and structures; some is relational, changing relationships between service users and academics, or service users and practitioners; some is about changing identity, how people see themselves, how others see them – challenging previous stigma and stereotypes. Effectively, this ought to be empowering and emancipatory for all concerned: staff and service users. The reality is imperfect, having some of these features some of the time. Service users and carers state they wish to 'make a difference'. This might involve transformations of academia, tutorial staff and researchers' attitudes and behaviour, practitioner behaviour, whole services, personal identities, or personal confidence and empowerment. All of these things are open to big or small changes – but sometimes the smallest change can have quite profound effects.

The struggle is to maximise the potential for authentic empowerment and change. To achieve this, interesting forms of organisation can occur within the service user/carer group (in our case the Community Involvement Team, CIT). People take care to organise themselves according to shared values and principles. They respect each other, work hard at consensus decision making, and accommodate the pace of the slowest. Within the CIT there is a division of labour playing to group members' talents and strengths, but everyone can take on any role, without being constrained by consideration of hierarchy.

In one sense, the idea of service user involvement within universities is a bureaucratic phenomenon, with the potential for box ticking and superficiality. Authentic involvement is something else. The fact that this is on personal and institutional agendas is arguably because of campaigning by service users and carers themselves, with the support of key academic and practitioner allies. Even if we suspect a degree of cynicism in the promotion of user involvement, we can take advantage of the opportunities presented.

In many ways Comensus mirrors this. Arguably, we got the start-up money and have been able to defend ourselves because of national and institutional commitments, but there has also been significant genuine support from various managers and academics. It is a good thing to be high on the agenda, but this should not detract from the implicit value of involvement and should also highlight a healthy suspicion towards attempts at incorporation or lip service.

A big challenge is the clash between a standing culture that privileges academic knowledge and expertise over and above outsider knowledge, for example service users or carers. Factors such as language, occupational closure, vanity and arrogance, narrow professional identity and mystique of science can work on different levels to exclude lay people from participation. Obviously, this can be a matter of degree, and it is possible that the newer universities are less hung up in this regard. If we consider this in terms of access to research participation, however, at all stages of the research process, up to and including user led research, there is clearly a long road to travel. Despite various funding councils stating a commitment to user involvement in research and bids being rated for how they address this, the same high ranked universities still garner most of the available funding.

In some instances, a perceived 'split' between academics and service user/carers may be blurred at the personal level. This may be because of shared personal experiences of service use, history of resistance in services in a previous life as practitioner, or academics may hold various political allegiances or values which can lead them to be internal 'activists' for institutional change. Integration at a strategic level is much greater now than when we started but still could be improved. Strategic influence at the top table is still limited, however, suggesting efforts towards culture change need to continue.

The structures we have developed within Comensus are effective and appreciated, but there is still a need to get more individual academics thoroughly engaged and inputting with time and effort. We also need to think about external links as much as internal – for example, local community and wider communities of interest and practice. These include connections with initiatives in other universities, supportive networks such as DUCIE (Developers of User and Carer Involvement in Education) and mhhe (Mental Health in Higher Education), but also the wider service user movement, trade unions and international links.

Roles, Identities and Rewards

Some academics who have been involved from the start have seen their role change to become more closely engaged in supporting service user and carer involvement. Institutional pressures mean that these commitments are not always fully acknowledged as an appropriate use of time, but academic roles can be sufficiently flexible to accommodate these changes. Other academics with heavier teaching commitments are not so fortunate. There are many pressures on contemporary academics, and the willing horses can tend to be flogged. Various factors are complicit in diminishing the autonomy of academics to dictate how their work is best organised (research and teaching quality assessment, governmental policies for involvement, need for grant capture, project management, targets, individual appraisal, etc.). Worsening conditions for students in the economy arguably lead to increasing demands for pastoral support too, and can increase the load of emotional labour. Conversely, for academics, being closely involved in service user and carer initiatives can be a key factor in job fulfilment and having a positive disposition towards work.

Our very identity can be at stake amidst the work of involvement: how people see themselves and how they are seen by others is open to transformation. Authentic engagement can afford practitioner educators an opportunity to re-connect with some of the values and motivations important in bringing them into the job in the first place. This positive sense of self as a practitioner can be threatened by various forms of alienation found in services which arise from conflict-laden relationships with service users; contradicting a sense of how staff may wish to see themselves as caring and kind individuals. Our experiences suggest that alliances with service users and carers offer the potential to achieve redemption from this sorry state of affairs, and university classrooms and research projects are uniquely situated to bring this about, to the benefit of all.

Academic staff involved with Comensus, and with many other engagement schemes from a range of countries, report becoming better at relationships with participants and behaving more inclusively in meetings and other scholarly activity such as research and writing. For those academics most closely involved, they inescapably experience, alongside people, emotions connected to work in the university and their lives away from the university: aspirations, frustrations, irritations, anger, sadness, anxiety and, of course, receive kindnesses and warmth from people too, sharing their happiness and satisfaction at jobs well done. Some of this was brought into stark relief by the death in a car accident of our first coordinator, Eileen, relatively early on in the project, and two recent deaths of valued members of the CIT, Les Collier and Lillian Hughes. The impact of these sad and tragic events has worked to strengthen solidarity and relationships in the group. We are all agreed that the quality of relationships between participants is one of the real strengths of Comensus.

Some of the teaching sessions delivered by service users have been without a doubt a privilege to be part of. These have involved truly profound connections between sensitive personal disclosure and the learning needs of students. There has also been the odd 'epiphany' moment, where individuals have become acutely aware of the profundity of their contribution, appreciated the impact of this on the respective audience, or begun to feel the shift in power towards a more valued identity or self-image. Invariably, all of this is personally affirming and gratifying in terms of knowledge that one has contributed to supporting this to happen; usually this is implicit but quite often direct compliments and thanks are expressed and reciprocated – all of these things keep us going.

Securing the Future

There is a powerful case to be made for service user and carer involvement in higher education, and for the need to avoid tokenism and to strive for authenticity.

Authenticity and action comprise an interesting couple: authenticity begets action and, in action, authenticity can be realised. We hope this book has emphasised the need for a systematic and integrated approach to involvement as opposed to piecemeal developments. As our text indicates, there is dissonance at a number of levels between the rhetoric of engagement, and the reality of resistance to the consequences of power-sharing, and of loss of expert status amongst professionals, both staff and students. As Chapters 8 and 10 illustrated explicitly, 'service users and carers' did not offer one homogenous party line on the range of problems and challenges implicit in engagement processes. This was also true of health and social care professionals, and of education staff. There were a wide range of interests, beliefs, conflicts and disagreements within and between individuals and groups in the engagement arena. This was a positive factor that generated creativity and the potential for unexpected emergence. It should be nurtured and not suppressed by a simplifying movement towards assigning people to a 'service user' position, or to a 'healthcare staff' position.

Throughout the book, we have noted numerous barriers to effective and authentic engagement. These included the terminology that was used; the accessibility of universities to service users; payment issues; and the problem of sustaining engagement projects that are set up with short-term funding. We have also identified factors for success in this endeavour. These included clear and agreed definitions for success, and regular and appropriate assessment of movement towards these goals; planning, horizon scanning and being open to emergence; and keeping faith with the ideology of engagement, by looking beyond fashionable policy and towards a shared vision of what is best in the long run. Ultimately, we strongly believe that this can be achieved most naturally if those working towards engagement are authentically motivated towards the achievement of optimum well-being for all of those involved. This requires shared values, courage, trust and cultural humility.

The involvement agenda for universities concerned with the education of future generations of practitioners and associated research mirrors similar imperatives within services themselves and the wider fora of policy formulation, governance and government. We contend that there are differences in effecting change within a university as opposed to the clinical practice arena. Both are a challenge, but arguably it can be easier in a university because those of us from practitioner backgrounds are not held responsible by our service user and carer colleagues for experiences of failings in care (rightly or wrongly). This creates the space for trust to develop through shared endeavour towards common goals, sustaining alliances and boosting solidarity between participants, whatever their personal background. If we are to be successful we have to work in alliance, have a shared value base and be committed to drive the process forward, even (or especially) when this seems to be in the face of organizational or individual resistance.

The altruistic bringing forward of personal experiences as a contribution to teaching and learning is a real gift to universities and the students within them. It is the task of all of us to support this as much as benefit from it.

References

Antonovsky, A. (1987) *Unravelling the Mystery of Health – How People Manage Stress and Stay Well*, Jossey-Bass Publishers, San Francisco.

Antonovsky, A. (1993) The implications of salutogenesis: an outsiders view, in *Cognitive Coping, Families and Disability* (eds A.P. Turnbull, J.M. Patterson, S.K. Behr *et al.*), Paul H Brookes, Baltimore.

Arnstein, S. (1969) A ladder of citizen participation. *Journal of the American Institute of Planners*, **35**, 216–224.

Ashcraft, M. (2007) Community consensus building: process management techniques (and strategies). *Public Management*, **89**(11), 16–18.

Ball, W. (2005) From community engagement to political engagement. *Political Science and Politics*, **38**, 287–291.

Barker, C. (2001) Fear, laughter and collective power: the making of Solidarity at the Lenin shipyard in Gdansk, Poland, August 1980, in *Passionate Politics* (eds J. Goodwin, J. Jasper and F. Poletta), University of Chicago Press, Chicago, pp. 175–194.

Barker, C. and Cox, L. (2002) *"What have the Romans Ever Done for Us?"* Academic and Activist Theorizing. Proceedings of 8th Annual Alternative Futures and Popular Protest Conference, Manchester Metropolitan University, Manchester. Available at: http://eprints.nuim.ie/428/ (accessed 23 July 2009).

Barley, G.E., Fisher, J., Dwinnell, B. and White, K. (2006) Teaching foundational physical examination skills: study results comparing lay teaching associates and physician instructors. *Academic Medicine*, **81**, 595–597.

Barnes, D., Carpenter, J. and Bailey, D. (2000) Partnerships with service users in interprofessional education for community mental health: a case study. *Journal of Interprofessional Care*, **14**(2), 189–200.

Barnes, M. and Morris, K. (2007) Networks, connectedness and resilience: learning from the Children's Fund in context. *Social Policy and Society*, **6**(2), 193–197.

Bar-On, R. (2006) The Bar-On model of emotional-social intelligence (ESI). *Psicothema*, **18**(suppl.), 13–25.

Barr, A. (2005) The contribution of research to community development. *Community Development Journal*, **40**, 453–458.

Barr, H., Koppel, I., Reeves, S. *et al.* (2005) *Effective Inter-Professional Education: Argument, Experience and Evidence*, Blackwell Publishing, Oxford.

Barton, L. (ed.) (2001) *Disability Politics and the Struggle for Change*, David Fulton, London.

Barton, M.B., Morley, D.S., Moore, S. *et al.* (2004) Decreasing women's anxieties after abnormal mammograms: a controlled trial. *Journal of the National Cancer Institute*, **96**, 529–538.

Basaglia, F. (1987) *Psychiatry Inside Out: Selected Writings of Franco Basaglia* (eds N. Scheper-Hughes and A.M. Lovell), Columbia University Press, New York.

Bayley, C. (2006) Community bridge building. *U (Unison members' magazine)*, New Year issue, 12–14.

Basset, T. (1999) Involving service users in training. *CARE: The Journal of Practice and Development*, **7**, 5–11.

Basset, T., Campbell, P. and Anderson, J. (2006) Service user/survivor involvement in mental health training and education: overcoming the barriers. *Social Work Education*, **25**, 393–402.

Batson, C., Ahmad, N. and Tsang, J. (2002) Four motives for community involvement. *Journal of Social Issues*, **58**, 429–445.

Beaton, B.E. and Clark, J.P. (2009) Qualitative research: a review of methods with use of examples from the total knee replacement literature. *Journal of Bone and Joint Surgery (American Edition)*, **91**(Suppl. 3), 107–112.

Bell, T. (2001) Imagining marketopia. *Dissent*, **48**(3), 74–80.

Benner, P. (1984) *From Novice to Expert: Excellence and Power in Clinical Nursing Practice*, Addison-Wesley, Menlo Park, CA.

Beresford, P. (2005a) 'Service user': regressive or liberatory terminology? *Disability & Society*, **20**, 469–477.

Beresford, P. (2005b) Theory and practice of user involvement in research, in *Involving Service Users in Health and Social Care Research* (eds L. Lowes and I. Hulatt), Routledge, Abingdon, pp. 6–17.

Beresford, P. and Campbell, J. (1994) Disabled people, service users, user involvement and representation. *Disability & Society*, **9**, 315–325.

Beresford, P., Branfield, F., Taylor, J. *et al.* (2006) Working together for better social work education. *Social Work Education*, **25**, 326–331.

Beuchler, S. (2000) *Social Movements in Advanced Capitalism*, Oxford University Press, Oxford.

Bevis, E. and Murray, J. (1990) The essence of the curriculum revolution: emancipatory teaching. *Journal of Nursing Education*, **29**, 326–331.

Birchall, J. (1997) *The International Co-operative Movement*, Manchester University Press, Manchester.

Bland, C.J., Starnaman, S., Harris, D. *et al.* (2000) "No fear" curricular change: monitoring curricular change in the W. K. Kellogg Foundation's national initiative on community partnerships and health professions education. *Academic Medicine*, **75**, 623–633.

Bland, C.J., Starnaman, S., Hembroff, L. *et al.* (1999) Leadership behaviors for successful university–community collaborations to change curricula. *Academic Medicine*, **74**, 1227–1237.

Blumer, H. (1969) *Symbolic Interactionism: Perspective and Method*, Prentice-Hall, Englewood Cliffs, NJ.

Bode, B.H. (1929) *Conflicting Psychologies of Learning*, DC Heath and Company, Lexington, MA.

Bolton, S. (2001) Changing faces: nurses as emotional jugglers. *Sociology of Health and Illness*, **23**(1), 85–100.

Bond, L., Holmes, T., Byrne, C. *et al.* (2008) Movers and shakers: how and why women become and remain engaged in community leadership. *Psychology of Women Quarterly*, **32**, 48–64.

Bourdieu, P. (1977) *Outline of a Theory of Practice* (ed. trans. R. Nice), Cambridge University Press, Cambridge.

Bourdieu, P. (1986) Forms of capital, in *Handbook of Theory and Research for the Sociology of Education* (ed. J. Richardson), Greenwood, New York, pp. 241–258.

Boyer, E.L. (1990) *Scholarship Reconsidered: Priorities of the Professoriate*, Carnegie Foundation for the Advancement of Teaching, Princeton, NJ.

Bradshaw, P. (2008) Service user involvement in the NHS in England: genuine user participation or a dogma-driven folly? *Journal of Nursing Management*, **16**, 673–681.

Bramble, T. and Minns, J. (2005) Whose streets? Our streets! Activist perspectives on the
Australian anti-capitalist movement. *Social Movement Studies*, **4**(2), 105–121.

Branch, V.K. and Lipsky, P.E. (1998) Positive impact of an intervention by arthritis educators on retention of information, confidence, and examination skills of medical students.
Arthritis Care and Research, **11**, 32–38.

Branch, V.K., Graves, G., Hanczyc, M. and Lipsky, P.E. (1999) The utility of trained arthritis
patient educators in the evaluation and improvement of musculoskeletal examination
skills of physicians in training. *Arthritis Care and Research*, **12**, 61–69.

Branfield, F. and Shaping Our Lives (2007) User Involvement in Social Work Education,
Social Care Institute for Excellence, London.

Branfield, F., Beresford, P. and Levin, E. (2007) Common Aims: A Strategy to Support
Service User Involvement in Social Work Education, Social Care Institute for Excel-
lence/Shaping Our Lives, London.

British Psychological Society (2008) *Good Practice Guidelines: Service User and Carer Involvement within Clinical Psychology Training*, BPS, Leicester.

Brown, A. (1998) *Organisational culture*, 2nd edn, Pitman, London.

Brown, P. and Zavetoski, S. (2005) Social movements in health: an introduction, in *Social
Movements in Health* (eds P. Brown and S. Zavetoski), Blackwell Publishing, Oxford, pp.
1–16.

Broyard, A. (1992) *Intoxicated by My Illness and Other Writings on Life and Death*, Ballantine
Books, New York.

Burgmann, V. (2003) *Power, Profit and Protest: Australian Social Movements and Globalisation*,
Allen and Unwin, Crows Nest, Australia.

Burrows, G. (2004) In whose interest. *New Statesman*, **133**(Feb 9), 28.

Burton, M. and Kagan, C. (2007) The creation of settings as social change: the role of social
movements. http://www.compsy.org.uk/CPSOCM2.PDF (accessed 9 January 2010).

Buttle, M. (2008) Diverse economies and the negotiations and practices of ethical finance:
the case of Charity Bank. *Environment and Planning A*, **40**, 2097–2113.

Calderon, J. (2004) Lessons from an activist intellectual: participatory research, teaching and
learning for social change. *Latin American Perspectives*, **31**, 81–94.

Campbell, P. (1996) The history of the user movement in the United Kingdom, in *Mental
Health Matters: A Reader* (eds T. Heller, J. Reynolds, R. Gomm *et al.*). Macmillan in association with the Open University, Basingstoke.

Campbell, P. (2005) From little acorns: the mental health service user movement, in *Beyond
the Water Towers: The Unfinished Revolution in Mental Health Services 1985–2005* (eds A. Bell
and P. Lindley), Sainsbury Centre for Mental Health, London.

Campbell, P. (2009) The service user/survivor movement, in *Mental Health Still Matters*
(eds J. Reynolds, R. Muston, T. Heller *et al.*), Open University/Palgrave Macmillan,
Houndmills.

Campbell, P. and Lindow, V. (1997) *Changing Practice: Mental Health Nursing and User
Empowerment*, Royal College of Nursing Learning Materials/MIND, London.

Campbell, P. and Roberts, A. (2009) Survivors' history. *A Life in the Day*, **13**, 3, 34–36.

Campbell, D.T. and Stanley, J.C. (1963) *Experimental and Quasi-Experimental Designs for
Research*, Rand McNally & Co, Chicago.

Campus Compact (2009) Campus Compact website: www.compact.org (accessed 29 April
2009).

Cannon, R. and Newble, D. (2000) *A Handbook for Teachers in Universities and Colleges: A Guide for Improving Teaching Methods*, 4th edn, Kogan Page, London.

Carey, M. (2009) 'It's a bit like being a robot or working in a factory': does Braverman help explain the experiences of state social workers in Britain since 1971. *Organization*, **16**, 505–527.

Carr, S. (2008) Personalisation A Rough Guide (Report 20), Social Care Institute for Excellence, London.

Carr, W. and Kemmis, S. (1986) *Becoming Critical: Education, Knowledge and Action Research*, Fabian, London.

Carty, V. and Onyett, J. (2006) Protest, cyberactivism and new social movements: the re-emergence of the peace movement post 9/11. *Social Movement Studies*, **5**(3), 229–249.

Castells, M. (1996) *The Information Age Vol 1: The Rise of the Network Society*, Blackwell Publishing, Oxford.

Castells, M. (1997) *The Information Age Vol 2: The Power of Identity*, Blackwell Publishing, Oxford.

Castells, M. (1998) *The Information Age Vol 3: End of Millenium*, Blackwell Publishing, Oxford.

Chell, E. (2007) Social enterprise and entrepreneurship: towards a convergent theory of the entrepreneurial process. *International Small Business Journal*, **25**(1), 5–26.

Church, K. (1995) Yes We Can! Promote Economic Opportunity and Choice Through Community Business, Ontario Council of Alternative Businesses, Toronto.

Church, K. (1996) *Forbidden Narratives: Critical Autobiography as Social Science*, Routledge, London.

Church, K. (1997) Because of Where We've Been. The Business Behind the Business of Psychiatric Survivor Economic Development, Ontario Council of Alternative Businesses, Toronto.

Church, K. (2005) Conflicting knowledge/s: user involvement in the field of knowledge, in *Field of Knowledge of Psychiatric and Mental Health Nursing* (ed. S. Tilley), Blackwell, London, pp. 181–185.

Church, K. (2006a) Working like crazy on 'Working Like Crazy:' Imag(in)ing CED practice through documentary film, in *Community Economic Development: Building for Social Change* (ed. E. Shragge), University College of Cape Breton, pp. 169–182.

Church, K. (2006b) Consumer-run businesses, in *Encyclopedia of Disability* (ed. G. Albrecht), Sage, Thousand Oaks, CA, pp. 312–316.

Church, K. (2008a) Exhibiting as inquiry: travels of an accidental curator, in *Handbook of the Arts in Qualitative Social Science Research* (eds A. Cole and J.G. Knowles), Sage, Thousand Oaks, CA, pp. 421–434.

Church, K. (2008b) The turbulence of learning to publish, in *Learning through Community: Exploring Participatory Practices* (eds K. Church, N. Bascia and E. Shragge), Springer Science and Business Media, B.V., Amsterdam, pp. v–vii.

Church, K., Bascia, N. and Shragge, E. (2008) The turbulence of academic collaboration, in *Learning Through Community: Exploring Participatory Practices* (eds K. Church, N. Bascia and E. Shragge), Springer Science and Business Media, B.V., pp. 3–20.

Church, K., Shragge, E., Fontan, J. and Ng, R. (2008) While no-one is watching: learning in social action among people who are excluded from the labour market, in *Learning Through Community: Exploring Participatory Practices* (eds K. Church, N. Bascia and E. Shragge), Springer Science and Business Media, B.V., pp. 97–115.

Chur-Hanson, A. and Koopowitz, L. (2004) The patient's voice in a problem-based learning case. *Australian Psychiatry* **12**(1), 31–35.

City University London (2006) User and Carer Involvement in Educational Activity, St Bartholomew School of Nursing and Midwifery, City University, London. http://www.city.ac.uk/sonm/mhld/involving_users/guidelines.html (accessed 9 January 2010).

Coates, D. (1990) Traditions of thought and the rise of social science in the United Kingdom, in *Society and Social Science: A Reader* (eds J. Anderson and M. Ricci), The Open University, Milton Keynes.

Cohen, G. (1995) *Self-Ownership, Freedom and Equality*, Cambridge University Press, Cambridge.

Cohen, J. (1985) Strategy or identity: new theoretical paradigms and contemporary social movements. *Social Research*, **52**, 663–716.

Cohen, J. (2007) Viewpoint: linking professionalism to humanism: what it means, why it matters. *Academic Medicine*, **82**(11), 1029–1032.

Coleman, E.A., Parry, C., Chalmers, S. and Min, S. (2006) The care transitions intervention: Results of a randomized controlled trial. *Archives of Internal Medicine*, **166**, 1822–1828.

Colliver, J.A. and McGaghie, W.C. (2008) The reputation of medical education research: quasi-experimentation and unresolved threats to validity. *Teaching and Learning in Medicine*, **20**, 101–103.

Colliver, J.A., Kucera, K. and Verhust, S.J. (2008) Meta-analysis of quasi-experimental research. *Medical Education*, **42**, 858–865.

Comensus Advisory Group (2004) Terms of Reference, Comensus, University of Central Lancashire, Preston.

Cone, D. and Payne, P. (2002) When campus and community collide: campus–community partnerships from a community perspective. *The Journal of Public Affairs*, **6**(supplemental issue 1), 203–218.

Cook, R. (2006) What does social enterprise mean for community nursing. *British Journal of Community Nursing*, **11**(11), 472–474.

Cooper, H. and Spencer-Dawe, E. (2006) Involving service users in interprofessional education narrowing the gap between theory and practice. *Journal of Interprofessional Care*, **20**, 603–617.

Cooper, H., Braye, S. and Geyer, R. (2004) Complexity and interprofessional education. *Learning in Health and Social Care*, **3**(4), 179–189.

Cooperrider, D.L. and Srivastva, S. (1987) Appreciative inquiry in organizational life, in *Research in Organization Change and Development*, vol. **1** (eds W. Pasmore and R. Woodman), JAI Press, Greenwich, CT.

Cooperrider, D.L., Sorensen, P.F., Whitney, D. and Yaeger, T.F. (eds) (2000) *Appreciative Inquiry*, Stipes Publishing LLC, Champaign, IL.

Corbin, J. and Strauss, A. (2008) *Basics of Qualitative Research*, 3rd edn, Sage, London.

Cornelius, N., Todres, M., Janjuha-Jivraj, S. *et al.* (2008) Corporate social responsibility and the social enterprise. *Journal of Business Ethics*, **81**, 355–370.

Coser, R. (1963) Alienation and the social structure: case analysis of a hospital, in *The Hospital in Modern Society* (ed. E. Friedson), Collier-Macmillan Ltd, London.

Costello, J. and Horne, M. (2001) Patients as teachers? An evaluative study of patients' involvement in classroom teaching. *Nurse Education in Practice*, **1**, 94–102.

Cott, C. (1998) Structure and meaning in multidisciplinary teamwork, *Sociology of Health and Illness*, **20**(6), 848–873.

Cottingham, A.H., Suchman, A.L., Litzelman, D.K. *et al.* (2008) Enhancing the informal curriculum of a medical school: a case study in organizational culture change. *Journal of General Internal Medicine*, **23**, 715–722.

Coupland, K., Davis, E. and Gregory, K. (2001) Learning from life. *Mental Health Care*, **4**, 166–169.

Cox, P. (2009) 'Connectivity': seeking conditions and connections for radical discourses and praxes in health, mental health and social work. *Social Theory and Health*, **7**, 170–186.

Cox, P., Geisen, T. and Green, R. (2008) Introduction, in *Qualitative Research and Social Change: European Contexts*, Palgrave Macmillan, Basingstoke.

Cox, L. and Fominaya, C. (2009) Editorial. Movement knowledge: what do we know, how do we create knowledge, and what do we do with it? *Interface*. (open access journal) http://www.interfacejournal.net/2009/01/issue-one-editorial-movement-knowledge. html (accessed 7 January 2010)

Cranford, C. and Ladd, D. (2003) Community unionism: organising for fair employment in Canada. *Just Labour*, **3**(Fall), 46–59.

Cranton, P. (1994) *Understanding and Promoting Transformative Learning: A Guide for Educators of Adults*, Jossey-Bass, San Francisco, CA.

Coleman, J. (1988) Social capital in the creation of human capital. *American Journal of Sociology*, **94** (Suppl.), s95–s120.

Crawford, M. (2001) Involving users in the development of psychiatric services – No longer an option, *Psychiatric Bulletin*, **22**(3), 155–157.

Crawford, M., Rutterm, D., Manley, C. *et al.* (2002) Systematic review of involving patients in the planning and development of health care. *British Medical Journal*, **325**, 1263–1265.

Crepaz-Keay, D., Binns, D. and Wilson, E. (1997) *Dancing with Angels – Involving Survivors in Mental Health Training*, CCETSW, London.

Cresswell, M. (2005) "Silent screams": Deliberate Self-Harm and the "Pathologised" Body. First International Conference Community, Work and Family: Change and Transformation, Manchester Metropolitan University, Manchester, 16–18 March 2006.

Cresswell, M. and Spandler, H. (2009) Psychopolitics: Peter Sedgwick's legacy for the politics of mental health. *Social Theory and Health*, **7**, 129–147.

Crossley, N. (1999a) Fish, field, habitus and madness: the first wave mental health users movement. *British Journal of Sociology*, **50**(4), 647–670.

Crossley, N. (1999b) Working utopias and social movements: an investigation using case study materials from radical mental health movements in Britain. *Sociology*, **33**, 809–830.

Crossley, N. (2002) *Making Sense of Social Movements*, Open University Press, Buckingham.

Crossley, N. (2006) *Contesting psychiatry: social movements in mental health*, Routledge, London.

Crossley, N. and Roberts, J.M. (eds) (2004) *After Habermas: New Perspectives on the Public Sphere*, Blackwell Publishing, Oxford.

Dart, R. (2004) The legitimacy of social enterprise. *Nonprofit Management and Leadership*, **14**, 411–424.

Dammers, J., Spencer, J., and Thomas, M. (2001) Using real patients in problem-based learning: students' comments on the value of using real, as opposed to paper cases, in a problem-based learning module in general practice. *Medical Education*, **35**, 27.

Davies, C. (1995) *Gender and the Professional Predicament in Nursing*, Open University Press, Milton Keynes.

Davies, W. and Herbert, D. (1993) *Communities Within Cities: An Urban Social Geography*, Belhaven Press, London.

Davidson, R., Duerson, M., Rathe, R. *et al.* (2001) Using standardized patients as teachers: a concurrent controlled trial. *Academic Medicine*, **76**, 840–843.

Day, R. (2005) *Gramsci is Dead: Anarchist Currents in the Newest Social Movements*, Pluto Press, London.

Deal, T. and Kennedy, A. (1982) *Corporate Cultures: The Rites and Rituals of Corporate Life*, Addison-Wesley, Reading, MA.

Deber, R., Kraetschmer, N., Urowitz, S. and Sharpe, N. (2005) Patient, consumer, client, or customer: what do people want to be called? *Health Expectations*, **8**, 345–351.

Delanty, G. (2003) *Community*. Routledge, London.

De Leonardis, O. and Mauri, D. (1992) From deinstitutionalisation to the social enterprise. *Social Policy*, **23**(2), 50–54.

Della Porta, D. and Diani, M. (2006) *Social Movements: An Introduction*, 2nd edn, Blackwell Publishing, Oxford.

de Tocqueville, A. (1966) *Democracy in America* (eds J. Mayer and M. Lerner, trans. G. Lawrence), Harper and Row, New York.

DH (Department of Health) (1994a) Implementing Caring for People, 'It's our lives', Community Care for People with Learning Disabilities, Department of Health, London.

DH (Department of Health) (1994b) Working in Partnership: Review of Mental Health Nursing, HMSO, London.

DH (Department of Health) (1998b) A First Class Service: Quality in the New NHS, Department of Health, London.

DH (Department of Health) (1998a) Modernising Social Services, Department of Health, London.

DH (Department of Health) (2000a) The NHS Plan, HMSO, London.

DH (Department of Health) (2000b) Delivering the NHS Plan: Next Steps on Investment – Next Steps on Reform, Department of Health, London.

DH (Department of Health) (2001a) Involving Patients and the Public in Healthcare: A Discussion Document, Department of Health, London.

DH (Department of Health) (2001b) The Expert Patient: A New Approach to Chronic Disease Management for the 21st Century, HMSO, London.

DH (Department of Health) (2002b) Listening, Hearing and Responding: Core Principles for the Involvement of Children and Young People, Department of Health, London.

DH (Department of Health) (2002a) Requirements for the Degree in Social Work, Department of Health, London.

DH (Department of Health) (2003) Streamlining Quality Assurance in Healthcare Education, Department of Health, London.

DH (Department of Health) (2004a) NHS Improvement Plan: Putting People at the Heart of Public Services, Department of Health, London.

DH (Department of Health) (2004b) Patient and Public Involvement in Health: The Evidence for Policy Implementation, Department of Health, London.

DH (Department of Health) (2005) Creating a Patient led NHS: Delivering the NHS Improvement Plan, Department of Health, London.

DH (Department of Health) (2006c) A Stronger Local Voice. A Framework for Creating a Stronger Local Voice in the Development of Health and Social Care Services, Department of Health, London.

DH (Department of Health) (2006b) From Values to Action: The Chief Nursing Officers Review of Mental Health Nursing, Department of Health, London.

DH (Department of Health) (2006a) Our Health Our Care Our Say: A New Direction for Community Services, HMSO, London.

DH (Department of Health) (2007) Putting People First: A Shared Vision and Commitment to the Transformation of Adult Social Care, Department of Health, London.

DH (Department of Health) (2008) A High Quality Workforce. NHS Next Stage Review (the Darzi review), Department of Health, London.

DH (Department of Health) (2009a) Personal Health Budgets: First Steps, Department of Health, London.

DH (Department of Health) (2009b) The NHS Constitution, Department of Health, London.

Dixon, S. and Clifford, A. (2007) Ecopreneurship – a new approach to managing the triple bottom line. *Journal of Organisational Change Management*, **20**(3), 326–345.

Donati, P. (1992) Political discourse analysis, in *Studying Collective Action* (eds M. Diani and R. Eyerman), Sage, London, pp. 136–167.

Downe, S., Kingdon, C., Finlayson, K. *et al.* (2009) Hard to reach? Access to maternity services for 'vulnerable' women in the North West. Report for NHSNW. Available from the University of Central Lancashire, sdowne@uclan.ac.uk.

Downe, S., McKeown, M., Johnson, E., *et al.* (2007) The UCLan community engagement and service user support (Comensus) project: valuing authenticity making space for emergence. *Health Expectations*, **10**, 392–406.

Doyal, L. and Pennell, I. (1979) *The Political Economy of Health*, Pluto Press, London.

Driedger, D. (1989) *The Last Civil Rights Movement*, Hurst, London.

Dreyfus, R. and Dreyfus, S.E. (1986) *Mind Over Machine: The Power of Human Intuition and Expertise in the Era of the Computer*, Basil Blackwell, Oxford.

DTI (Department for Trade and Industry) (2002) Social Enterprise: A Strategy for Success, Department for Trade and Industry, London.

Ducci, G., Stentella, C. and Vulterini, P. (2002) The social enterprise in Europe: the state of the art. *International Journal of Mental Health*, **31**(3), 76–91.

Duxbury, J. and Ramsdale, S. (2007) Involving service users in educational assessment. *Nursing Times*, **103**(1), 30–31.

Economist (2005) Good for me, good for my party. *Economist*, **377**(26), 71–72.

Edwards, G. (2004) Habermas and social movements: what's 'new'? *The Sociological Review*, **52**(1), 113–130.

Edwards, G. (2007) Habermas, activism and acquiescence: Reactions to 'colonization' in uk trade unions. *Social Movement Studies*, **6**(2), 111–130.

Edwards, G. (2008) The 'lifeworld' as a resource for social movement participation and the consequences of its colonization. *Sociology*, **42**(2), 299–316.

Eraut, M. (1994) *Developing Professional Knowledge and Competence*, The Falmer Press, London.

ESRC (Economic and Social Research Council) (2009) The Impact of HEIs on regional economies. Available from: http://www.esrcsocietytoday.ac.uk/ESRCInfoCentre/research/collaborations/HEIs.aspx (accessed 14th August 2009).

Faculty of Health (2005) Major Review: Self Evaluation Document, Faculty of Health, University of Central Lancashire, Preston.

Fanon, F. (1967) *The Wretched of the Earth*, Penguin, Harmondsworth.

Farrell, C., Towle, A. and Godolphin, W. (2006) Where's the Patient Voice in Health Professional Education? A Report from the 1st International Conference, Organized by the Division of Health Care Communication, College of Health Disciplines, University of British Columbia, Vancouver.

Fawcett, S., Fransisco, V. and Paine-Andrews, A. (2000) A model memorandum of collaboration: a proposal. *Public Health Reports*, **115**, 174–179.

Felton, A. and Stickley, T. (2004) Pedagogy, power and service user involvement. *Journal of Psychiatric and Mental Health Nursing*, **11**, 89–98.

Fink, A. and Kosecoff, J. (1985) *How to Conduct Surveys: A Step-By-Step Guide*, Sage, London.

Flanagan, J. (1999) Public participation in the design of educational programmes for cancer nurses: A case report. *European Journal of Cancer Care*, **8**, 107–112.

Flynn, F. and Chatman, J. (2001) Strong cultures and innovation: oxymoron or opportunity? in *Handbook of Organizational Cultures* (eds C. Cooper, C. Earley, J. Chatman and W. Starbuck), John Wiley & Sons, Ltd, Chichester.

Fountain, J., Patel, K. and Buffin, J. (2007) Community engagement: the Centre for Ethnicity and Health model, in *Overcoming Barriers: Migration, Marginalisation and Access to Health Services* (eds D. Domineg, J. Fountain, E. Schatz and G. Broring), Amsterdam Oecomenish Centrum (AOMC)/Correlation Network for Social Inclusion, Amsterdam.

Freeth, D., Hammick, M., Barr, H. *et al.* (2005) *Effective Interprofessional Education: Development, Delivery and Evaluation*, Blackwell, Oxford.

Freire, P. (1971) *Pedagogy of the Oppressed*, Herder & Herder, New York.

Freire, P. (1999) *Pedagogy of Hope: Reliving Pedagogy of the Oppressed*, Continuum, New York.

Froggett, L. and Chamberlayne, P. (2004) Narratives of social enterprise: from biography to practice and policy critique. *Qualitative Social Work*, **3**(1), 61–77.

Gecht, M.R. (2000) What happens to patients who teach. *Teaching and Learning in Medicine*, **12**, 171–175.

GMC (General Medical Council) (1993) Tomorrow's Doctors: Recommendations on Undergraduate Medical Education, GMC, London.

GSCC (General Social Care Council) (2005) Post-Qualifying Framework for Social Work Education and Training, GSCC, London.

GSCC/SCIE (General Social Care Council/Social Care Institute for Excellence) (2004) Living and Learning Together, SCIE, London.

Glaser, B.G. and Strauss, A.L. (1967) *The Discovery of Grounded Theory*, Aldine Publishing Company, New York.

Glassick, C.E. (2000a) Boyer's expanded definitions of scholarship, the standards for assessing scholarship and the elusiveness of the scholarship of teaching. *Academic Medicine*, **75**, 877–880.

Glassick, C.E. (2000b) Reconsidering scholarship. *Journal of Public Health Management and Practice*, **6**, 4–9.

Goffman, E. (1974) *Frame Analysis: An Essay in the Organization of Experience*, Harper and Row, New York.

Golding, S. (1992) *Gramsci's Democratic Theory – Contributions to a Post Liberal Democracy*, University of Toronto Press, Toronto.

Goss, S. and Miller, C. (1995) From Margin to Mainstream: User and Carer Centred Community Care, The Joseph Rowntree Foundation, York.

Gramsci, A. (1971) *Selections from the Prison Notebooks*, Lawrence and Wishart, London.

Greco, M., Brownlea, A. and McGovern, J. (2001) Impact of patient feedback on the interpersonal skills of general practice registrars: results of a longitudinal study. *Medical Education*, **35**, 748–756.

Green, S. (2007) *Involving People in Healthcare Policy and Practice*, Radcliffe Publishing, Seattle.

Greenhalgh, T. and Collard, A. (2003) *Narrative Based Healthcare: Sharing Stories - A Multiprofessional Workbook*, BMJ Books, London.

Guba, E.G. and Lincoln, Y.S. (1989) *Fourth Generation Evaluation*, Sage, London.

Gusfield, J. (1970) *Protest, Reform and Revolt*, John Wiley & Sons, Ltd, Chichester.

Haas, M. (1999) A critique of patient satisfaction. *Health Information Management*, **29**(1), 9–13.

Habermas, J. (1973) *Theory and Practice*, Beacon Press, Boston.

Habermas, J. (1976) *Legitimation Crisis*, Heinemann, London.

Habermas, J. (1981) New social movements. *Telos*, **49**(Fall), 33–37.

Hammick, M., Freeth, D., Goodsman, D. and Copperman, J. (2009) *Being Interprofessional*, Polity, Cambridge.

Hanifan L.J. (1916) The rural school community center. *Annals of the American Academy of Political and Social Science*, **67**, 130–138.

Hanley, B. (2005) Research as Empowerment? User Involvement in Research: Building on Experience and Developing Standards, Toronto Seminar Group/Joseph Rowntree Foundation, York.

Hanson, J.L. and Randall, V.F. (2007a) Advancing a partnership: patients, families and medical educators. *Teaching and Learning in Medicine*, **19**, 191–197.

Hanson, J.L. and Randall, V.F. (2007b) *Patients as Advisors: Enhancing Medical Education Curricula*, Uniformed Services University of the Health Sciences, Bethesda, MD.

Happell, B., Pinikahana, J. and Roper, C. (2002) Attitudes of postgraduate nursing students towards consumer participation in mental health services and the role of the consumer academic. *International Journal of Mental Health Nursing*, **11**, 240–250.

Haq, I., Fuller, J. and Dacre, J. (2006) The use of patient partners with back pain to teach undergraduate medical students. *Rheumatology*, **45**, 430–434.

Harding, R. (2007) Understanding social entrepreneurship. *Industry and Higher Education*, **21**(1), 73–84.

Hargadon, J. and Staniforth, M. (2000) A Health Service of all the Talents: Developing the NHS Workforce, Department of Health, London.

Harrison, N., Ingman, I., Moor, N. *et al.* (2006) Culture and processes in primary care, in *Enhancing Primary Care Mental Health Practice: An Interactive Teaching and Learning Resource for Practitioners Working with Common Mental Health Problems* (eds P. Myles and D. Rushforth), Trent WDC, Notts.

Haynes, D. and White, B. (1999) Will the real social work please stand up? A call to stand for professional unity. *Social Work*, **44**, 385–391.

Hays, R. (2007) Community activists' perceptions of citizenship roles in an urban community: a case study of attitudes that affect community engagement. *Journal of Urban Affairs*, **29**, 401–424.

Healy, K. (2000) *Social Work Practice: Contemporary Perspectives on Change*, Sage, London.

Healy, K. and Meagher, G. (2004) The reprofessionalisation of social work: collaborative approaches for achieving professional recognition. *British Journal of Social Work*, **34**, 243–260.

Hendry, G.D., Schrieber, L. and Bryce, D. (1999) Patients teach students: Partners in arthritis education. *Medical Education*, **33**, 674–677.

Hesse-Biber, S.N. and Leavy, P. (2008) *Emergent Methods*, Guilford Press, London.

Inui, T.S. and Frankel, R.M. (1991) Evaluating the quality of qualitative research: A proposal pro tem. *Journal of General Internal Medicine*, **6**, 485–486.

Higginson, I. and Carr, A. (2001) Measuring quality of life: using quality of life measures in the clinical setting. *British Medical Journal*, **322**, 1297–1300.

Hills, M. and Mullett, J. (2000) Community based research: creating evidence based change for health and social change. Paper presented at Qualitative Evidence Based Practice conference, Coventry University, 15–17 May 2000. Available at: http://www.leeds.ac.uk/educol/documents/00001388.htm (accessed 14th August 2009).

Health Life Sciences Partnership (2008) *Quality Assurance Handbook*, HLSP, Cambridge.

Hoefstede, G. (2001) *Culture's Consequences: Comparing Values, Behaviours, Institutions, and Organisations Across Nations*, 2nd edn, Sage, Thousand Oaks, California.

Hoerr, J. (1997) *We Can't Eat Prestige: The Women Who Organized Harvard*, Temple University Press, PA.

Holdsworth, C. and Quinn, J. (2006) HEIs and Local Communities: Forward and Backward Linkages: Report of an ESRC Network Project for Research Programme on the Impact of HEIs on Regional Economies. RES-171-25-0005, Economic and Social Research Council, London.

HM Government (2007) Putting People First: A Shared Vision and Commitment to the Transformation of Adult Social Care, HM Government, London.

Hyman, R. (2007) How can trade unions act strategically? *Transfer*, **13**(2), 193–210.

Ignagni, E. and Church, K. (2008) One more reason to look away? Ties and tensions between arts-informed inquiry and disability studies, in *Handbook of the Arts in Qualitative Social Science Research* (eds A. Cole and J.G. Knowles), Sage, Thousand Oaks, CA, pp. 625–638.

Involve (2006) A Guide to Reimbursing and Paying Members of the Public Who Are Actively Involved in Research, Department of Health, Eastleigh.

Involve (2007) Good Practice in Active Public Involvement in Research, Department of Health, Eastleigh.

Isaac, S. and Michael, W.B. (1995) *Handbook in Research and Evaluation for Education and the Behavioral Sciences*, 3rd edn, EdITS, San Diego.

Jacobs, J. (1961) *The Death and Life of Great American Cities*, Random House, New York.

Jacobson, M. and Zavos, A. (2007) Paranoia Network and conference: alternative communities and the disruption of pathology. *Journal of Critical Psychology, Counselling and Psychotherapy*, **7**, 28–39.

James, N. (1992) Care = organisation + physical labour + emotional labour. *Sociology of Health and Illness*, **14**(4), 488–509.

Jarley, P. (2005) Unions as social capital: renewal through a return to the logic of mutual aid? *Labor Studies Journal*, **29**(4), 1–26.

Jha, V., Quinton, N.D., Bekker, H.L. and Roberts, T.E. (2009a) Strategies and interventions for the involvement of real patients in medical education: A systematic review. *Medical Education*, **43**, 10–20.

Jha, V., Quinton, N.D., Bekker, H.L. and Roberts, T.E. (2009b) What educators and students really think about using patients as teachers in medical education: A qualitative study. *Medical Education*, **43**, 449–456.

Jones, L. (1994) *The Social Context of Health and Health Work*, Macmillan, Houndmills.

Jones, C., Ferguson, I., Lavalette, M. and Penketh, L. (2004) Social work and social justice: a manifesto for a new engaged practice. http://www.socmag.net/?p=177 (accessed 9 January 2010).

Kerlin, J. (2006) Social enterprise in the United States and Europe: understanding and learning from the differences. *Voluntas*, **17**, 247–263.

Kern, D.E., Thomas, P.A., Howard, D.M. and Bass, E.B. (1998) *Curriculum Development for Medical Education: A Six-step Approach*, The Johns Hopkins University Press, Baltimore.

Khoo, R., McVicar, A. and Brandon, D. (2004) Service user involvement in postgraduate mental health education. Does it benefit practice? *Journal of Mental Health*, **13**, 481–492.

Kirkpatrick, D.L. (1998) *Evaluating Training Programs: The Four Levels*, Berrett-Koehler Publishers, San Francisco.

Klandermans, B. (1997) *The Social Psychology of Protest*, Blackwell Publishers, Oxford.

Klein, N. (2002) *Fences and Windows: Dispatches from the Frontlines of the Globalization Debate*, Picador, Vintage, Canada.

Kline, R.B. (2009) *Becoming a Behavioral Science Researcher: A Guide to Producing Research that Matters*, Guilford Press, London.

Kohlberg, L. (1973) The claim to moral adequacy of a highest stage of moral judgment. *Journal of Philosophy*, **70**, 630–646.

Kohlberg, L. (1984) *Essays on Moral Development. Volume II. The Psychology of Moral Development*, Harper Row, New York.

Lathlean, J., Burgess, A., Coldham, T. *et al.* (2006) Experiences of service user and carer participation in health care. *Nurse Education Today*, **26**, 732–737.

Law, A. and Mooney, G. (2006) The maladies of social capital I: the missing 'capital' in theories of social capital. *Critique: Journal of Socialist Theory*, **34**(2), 127–143.

Leadbeater, C. (2002) Life in no mans land. *New Statesman*, **131** (June 3) (Suppl.), ii–iv.

Levin, E. (2004) Involving Service Users in Social Work Education, Resource Guide No. 2, Social Care Institute for Excellence, London.

Levin, K.S., Brauening, M.P., O'Malley, M.S. *et al.* (2000) Communicating results of diagnostic mammography: what do patients think? *Academic Radiology*, **7**, 1069–1076.

Levitas, R. (2004) Let's hear it for Humpty: social exclusion, the third way and cultural capital. *Cultural Trends*, **13**(2) No. 50, 1–15.

Lewin, K. (1946) Action research and minority problems. *Journal of Social Issues*, **2**(4), 34–46.

Lewis, J. (2009) Five things we need from a social investement bank. http://www.guardian.co.uk/society/joepublic/2009/jul/29/social-investment-bank appeared 29 July 2009 (accessed 30 July 2009).

Lincoln, Y.S. and Guba, E.G. (1985) *Naturalistic Inquiry*, Sage, London.

Littman, D. (2008) Another politics is possible. *Red Pepper*, 160 (June/July), 20–22.

Lowes, L. and Hulatt, I. (eds) (2005) *Involving Service Users in Health and Social Care Research*, Routledge, London.

Lown, B.A., Hanson, J.L. and Clark, W.D. (2009) Mutual influence in shared decision making: a collaborative study of patients and physicians. *Health Expectations*, **12**, 160–174.

Lown, B.A., Sasson, J.P. and Hinrichs, P. (2008) Patients as partners in radiology education: an innovative approach to teaching and assessing patient-centered communication. *Academic Radiology*, **15**, 425–432.

Luke, H. (2003) *Medical Education and Sociology of Medical Habitus: "It's not about the Stethoscope!"*, Kluwer Academic Publishers, Dordrecht, The Netherlands.

Lukes, S. (1984) Peter Sedgwick (1934–1983). *History Workshop Journal*, **17**(1), 211–213.

Magoon, A.J. (1977) Constructivist approaches in education research. *Review of Education Research*, **47**, 651–693.

Mancino, A. and Thomas, A. (2005) An Italian pattern of social enterprise: the social cooperative. *Nonprofit Management and Leadership*, **15**, 357–369.

Marks, L. and Hunter, J. (2007) Social Enterprise and the NHS: Changing Patterns of Ownership and Accountability, Unison, London.

Marris, P. (1982) *Community Planning and Conceptions of Change*, Routledge and Kegan Paul, London.

Marris, P. and Rein, M. (1967) *Dilemmas of Social Reform*, Penguin Books, Harmondsworth.

Maslow, A. (1994) *The Farther Reaches of Human Nature*, Penguin Compass, Arkana.

Mason, C., Kirkbride, J. and Bryde, D. (2007) From stakeholders to institutions: the changing face of social enterprise governance theory. *Management Decision*, **45**, 284–301.

Masters, H., Forrest, S., Harley, A. *et al.* (2002) Involving mental health service users and carers in curriculum development: moving beyond 'classroom' involvement. *Journal of Psychiatric and Mental Health Nursing*, **9**, 309–316.

Mayo, E. (2002) The dream and the reality. *New Statesman*, **131**(June 3) (Suppl.), xii–xii.

McLennan, D. (1977) *Karl Marx: Selected Writings*, Oxford University Press, Oxford.

McKeown, M. (1995) The transformation of nurses' work? *Journal of Nursing Management*, **3**(2), 67–74.

McKeown, M. (2009) Alliances in action: opportunities and threats to solidarity between workers and service users in health and social care disputes. *Social Theory and Health*, **7**, 148–169.

McKeown, M. and Spandler, H. (2006) Alienation and redemption: the potential for alliances with mental health service users. Paper presented at 11th International Alternative Futures and Popular Protest Conference, Manchester, 19–21 April 2006.

McNay, I. (ed.) (2000) *Higher Education and its Communities*, Open University Press, Milton Keynes.

Meads, G., Ashcroft, J., Barr, H. *et al.* (2005) *The Case for Interprofessional Collaboration in Health and Social Care*, Blackwell Publishing, Oxford.

Means, R. and Smith, R. (1998) *Community Care: Policy and Practice*, 2nd edn, Macmillan, Basingstoke.

Meegan, R. and Mitchell, A. (2001) 'It's not community round here, it's neighbourhood': neighbourhood change and cohesion in urban regeneration policies. *Urban Studies*, **38**, 2167–2194.

Melucci, A. (1996a) *The Playing Self: Person and Meaning in the Planetary Age*, Cambridge University Press, Cambridge.

Melucci, A. (1996b) *Challenging Codes: Collective Action in the Information Age*, Cambridge University Press, Cambridge.

Mental Health Recovery Study Working Group (2009) *Mental Health 'Recovery': Users and Refusers*, Wellesley Institute, Toronto.

Merriam, S.B. (1998) *Qualitative Research and Case Study Applications in Education*, Jossey-Bass, San Francisco.

Millers, L. and Walters, R. (2006) Redressing the Balance, MIND, Cymru, Wales.

Mills, G.E. (2000) *Action Research: A Guide for the Teacher Researcher*, Merrill (Prentice Hall), Columbus, OH.

Morgan, A. and Jones, D. (2009) Perceptions of service user and carer involvement in healthcare education and impact on students' knowledge and practice: a literature review. *Med Teach.*, **31**(2), 82–95.

Morrin, M., Simmonds, D. and Somerville, W. (2004) Social enterprise: mainstreamed from the margins? *Local Economy*, **19**(1), 69–84.

Morris, P., Armitage, A. and Symonds, J. (2005) Whose voice is it anyway? Embedding the patient voice in the simulated and standardized patient. Paper presented at the Where's the Patient Voice in Health Professional Education? 1st International Conference, University of British Columbia, Vancouver, CA. 3–5 November 2005.

MRC (Medical Research Council) (2008) Complex interventions guidance. Available at: http://www.mrc.ac.uk/Utilities/Documentrecord/index.htm?d=MRC004871 (accessed 14 August 2009).

National Board for Nursing and Midwifery for Scotland (2000) Fitness for Practice – Implementation in Scotland, NBS, Edinburgh.

NIH (National Institutes of Health) (2009) NCRR Fact Sheet: Clinical and Translational Science Awards, National Institutes of Health, US Department of Health and Human Services, Bethesda, Maryland, USA.

Neergaard, M.A., Olesen, F., Andersen, R.S. and Sondergaard, J. (2009) Qualitative description: The poor cousin of health research? *BMC Medical Research Methodology*, **9**, 52.

Newton, R.R. and Rudestam, K.E. (1999) *Your Statistical Consultant: Answers to Your Data Analysis Questions*, Sage, London.

NHS Executive (1999) Patient and Public Involvement in the New NHS, Department of Health, Leeds.

Northern Centre for Mental Health (2003) National Continuous Quality Improvement Tool for Mental Health Education, Northern Centre for Mental Health, York.

Nummenmaa, L., Hirvonen, J., Parkkola, R. and Hietanen, J. (2008) Is emotional contagion special? An fMRI study on neural systems for affective and cognitive empathy. *Neuroimage*, **43**(3), 571–580.

Nyssens, M. (ed.) (2006) *Social Enterprise: At the Crossroads of Market, Public Policies and Civil Society*, Routledge, London.

Ogbonna, E. (1992) Managing organizational culture: fantasy or reality? *Human Resource Management Journal*, **3**(2), 42–54.

Offe, C. (1985) New social movements: challenging the boundaries of institutional politics. *Social Research: an International Quarterly Journal of the Social Sciences*, **52**, 817–868.

Offe, C. (1987) Challenging the boundaries of institutional politics: social movements since the 1960s, in *Changing Boundaries of the Political: Essays in the Evolving Balance Between State and Society, Public and Private in Europe* (ed. C.S. Maier), Cambridge University Press, Cambridge, pp. 63–107.

Oliver, M. (1990) *The Politics of Disablement*, Macmillan, London.

O'Neill, F. (2002) Leeds Fitness for Practice Implementation: Developing a Strategic Approach to User and Carer Involvement in Pre-registration Nursing and Midwifery Education in Leeds, Leeds Metropolitan University, Leeds.

O'Toole, K. and Burdess, N. (2004) New community governance in small rural towns: the Australian experience. *Journal of Rural Studies*, **20**, 433–443.

Papadimitriou, T. (2007) A social experiment in the midst of G8 power: creating 'another world' or the politics of self-indulgence? Paper presented at 12th International Alternative Futures and Popular Protest Conference, Manchester, 2–4 April 2007.

Parkinson, C. and Howorth, C. (2008) The language of social entrepreneurs. *Entrepreneurship and Regional Development*, **20**, 285–309.

Panitch, M., Church, K. and Frazee, C. (2008) Out from Under: Disability, History and Things to Remember – The Exhibit Catalogue, Ryerson-RBC Institute for Disability Studies Research and Education, Toronto.

Parr, H. (2008) *Mental Health and Social Space: Towards Inclusionary Geographies*, Wiley-Blackwell, Oxford.

Paterniti, D., Pan, R., Smith, L. *et al.* (2006) From physician-centred to community-oriented perspectives on health care: assessing the efficacy of community based training. *Academic Medicine*, **81**(4), 347–353.

Pearce, J. (2003) *Social Enterprise in Anytown*, Calouste Gulbenkian Foundation, London.

Pearlin, L. (1962) Alienation from work: a study of nursing personnel. *American Sociological Review*, **27**, 314–326.

Pelias, R. (2004) *A Methodology of the Heart*, Altimira Press, Walnut Creek, CA.

Pennington, R. (2003) Change performance to change the culture. *Industrial and Commercial Training*, **35**, 251–255.

Pepin, J. (2005) Venture capitalists and entrepreneurs become venture philanthropists. *International Journal of Nonprofit Voluntary Sector Marketing*, **10**, 165–173.

Peters, T. and Waterman, R. (1982) *In Search of Excellence, Lessons from America's Best-Run Companies*, Harper and Row, New York.

Pheysey, D. (1993) *Organisational Cultures: Types and Transformations*, Routledge, London.

Phillips, M. (2006) Growing pains: the sustainability of social enterprises. *International Journal of Entrepreneurship and Innovation*, **7**, 221–231.

Pilgrim, D. (2005) Protest and co-option: the recent fate of the psychiatric patient's voice, in *Beyond the Water Towers: The Unfinished Revolution in Mental Health Services 1985–2005*, Sainsbury Centre for Mental Health, London.

Pilgrim, D. (2008) 'Recovery' and current mental health policy. *Chronic Illness*, **4**, 295–304.

Pitts, M. and Smith, A. (eds) (2007) *Researching the Margins: Strategies for Ethical and Rigorous Research with Marginalised Communities*, Palgrave Macmillan, Basingstoke.

Plsek, P. and Greenhalgh, T. (2001) The challenge of complexity in health care. *British Medical Journal*, **323**, 625–628.

Pliskin, J., Shepard, D. and Weinstein, M. (1980) Utility functions for life years and health status. *Operations Research* (Operations Research Society of America), **28**(1), 206–224.

Porter, S. (1998) *Social Theory and Nursing Practice*, Macmillan, Houndmills.

Powell, F. and Geoghegan, M. (2005) Reclaiming civil society: the future of global social work? *European Journal of Social Work*, **8**, 129–144.

Price, B. (2002) Social capital and factors affecting civic engagement as reported by leaders of voluntary associations. *The Social Science Journal*, **39**, 119–127.

Priest, S. (2001) A program evaluation primer. *Journal of Experiential Education*, **24**, 34–40.

Priestley, J., Hellawell, M. and McKeown, M. (2007) Building Bradton: actual experiences in a virtual world, collaborating with service users and carers to develop a virtual community. Paper presented at Service Improvement and Innovation in Health and Social Care (HEA/NHS Institute for Innovation and Improvement), 3 December 2007, York.

Public Administration Select Committee (2008) User Involvement in Public Services. HC 410, HMSO, London.

Putnam, R. (2000) *Bowling Alone: The Collapse and Revival of American Community*, Simon and Schuster, New York.

Race, P. (1999) Enhancing Student Learning, SEDA Special No 10, Staff and Educational Development Association (SEDA), London.

Race, P. and Brown, S. (2001) The ILTA Guide: Inspiring Learning about Teaching and Assessment, ILTA, York.

Raj, N., Badcock, I.J., Brown, G.A. *et al.* (2006) Undergraduate musculoskeeletal examination teaching by trained patient educators: A comparison with doctor-led teaching. *Rheumatology*, **45**, 1404–1408.

Rakel, D., Hoeft, T., Barrett, B. *et al.* (2009) Practitioner empathy and the duration of the common cold. *Family Medicine*, **41**, 494–501.

Randall, V.F. and Hanson, J.L. (2000) The family competency project. *Academic Medicine*, **75**, 529–530.

Rawlinson, J.W. (1990) Self awareness: conceptual influences, contribution to nursing, and approaches to attainment. *Nurse Education Today*, **10**, 111–117.

Raza, S., Rosen, M.P., Chorny, K. *et al.* (2001) Patient expectations and costs of immediate reporting of screening mammography. *American Journal of Roentgenology*, **177**, 579–583.

Rea, L.M. and Parker, R.A. (1997) *Designing and Conducting Survey Research: A Comprehensive Guide*, Jossey-Bass, San Francisco, CA.

Reason, P. and Bradbury, H. (eds) (2000) *Handbook of Action Research: Participative Inquiry and Practice*, Sage, London.

Repper, J. and Breeze, J. (2007) User and carer involvement in the training and education of health professionals: a review of the literature. *Journal of Nursing Studies*, **44**, 511–519.

Reynolds, J. and Read, J. (1999) Opening minds: user involvement in the production of learning materials on mental health and distress. *Social Work Education*, **18**, 417–431.

Richter, D., Gimarc, J. and Preston, G. (2003) Implementing community-campus partnerships in South Carolina: collaborative efforts to improve public health. *Public Health Reports*, **118**, 387–391.

Ridley-Duff, R. (2007) Communitarian perspectives on social enterprise. *Corporate Governance*, **15**(2), 382–392.

Robinson, F. (2009) Servant teaching: the power and promise for nursing education. *International Journal of Nursing Education Scholarship*, **6**(1), Article 5.

Robbins, S. (2001) *Organisational Behaviour*, 9th edn, Prentice-Hall, New Jersey.

Robert, G., Hardacre, J., Locock, L. *et al.* (2003) Redesigning mental health services: lessons on user involvement from the mental health collaborative. *Health Expectations*, **6**, 60–71.

Rogers, A. and Pilgrim, D. (1991) "Pulling down churches": accounting for the British mental health users movement. *Sociology of Health and Illness*, **13**(2), 129–148.

Rothschild, J. (2009) Workers cooperatives and social enterprise: a forgotten route to social equity and democracy. *American Behavioural Scientist*, **52**, 1023–1041.

Rothschild-Whitt, J. (1979) The collectivist organisation: an alternative to rational bureaucratic models. *American Sociological Review*, **44**, 509–526.

Rudman, M.J. (1996) User involvement in the nursing curriculum: Seeking users' views. *Journal of Psychiatric and Mental Health Nursing*, **3**, 195–200.

Ruta, D., Garratt, A. and Russell, I. (1999) Patient centred assessment of quality of life for patients with four common conditions. *Quality in Health Care*, **8**, 22–29.

Salovey, P. and Mayer, J.D. (1990) Emotional intelligence. *Imagination, Cognition, and Personality*, **9**, 185–211.

Salvage, J. (2002) *Rethinking Professionalism: The First Step for Patient Focused Care*, IPPR, London.

Saundry, R., Stuart, M. and Antcliff, V. (2008) Can social capital revitalise trade unions? An examination of worker networks in the UK audio-visual industries. Paper presented at BUIRA Annual Conference, University of the West of England, 26–28 June 2008.

Savan, B. (2004) Community–university partnerships: linking research and action for sustainable community development. *Community Development Journal*, **39**, 372–384.

Savin-Baden, M. (2000) *Problem-Based Learning in Higher Education: Untold Stories*, Open University Press/SRHE, Milton Keynes.

Savio, M. and Righetti, A. (1993) Cooperatives as social enterprise in Italy: a place for social integration and rehabilitation. *Acta Psychiatrica Scandinavica*, **88**, 238–242.

Sawley, L. (2002) Consumer groups: shaping education and developing practice. *Paediatric Nursing*, **14**, 18–21.

Schein, E. (1985) *Organizational Culture and Leadership*, Jossey Bass, San Fransisco.

Schensul, J.J. and Lecompte, M.D. (eds) (1999) *Ethnographer's Toolkit*, vol. **7**, Alta Mira Press, Walnut Creek, CA.

Scheyett, A. and Diehl, M. (2006) Walking our talk in social work education: partnering with consumers of mental health services. *Social Work Education*, **23**, 435–450.

Schofield, S. (2005) The case against social enterprise. *Journal of Cooperative Studies*, **38**(3), 34–39.

Schon, D. (1983) *The Reflective Practitioner: How Professionals Think in Action*, Temple Smith, London.

Sedgwick, P. (1982) *Psychopolitics*, Pluto Press, London.

Self, W. (2002) *Dorian: An Imitation*, Penguin, London.

SF36.org (2009) Available from: http://www.sf-36.org/tools/sf36.shtml (accessed 14 August 2009).

Shaw, E. (2004) Marketing in the social enterprise context: is it entrepreneurial? *Qualitative Market Research*, **7**(3), 194–205.

Simons, L., Tee, S., Lathlean, J. *et al.* (2007) A socially inclusive approach to user participation in higher education. JAN Original Research, Journal Compilation, Blackwell Publishing, London.

Simpson, A. (2006) Involving service users and carers in the education of mental health nurses. *Mental Health Practice*, **10**(4), 20–24.

Simpson, A. and Benn, L. (2007) Scoping Exercise to Inform the Development of a National Mental Health Carer Support Curriculum, City University, London.

Simpson, A. and Reynolds, L. (2008) Consulting the experts. *OpenMind*, **152**, 18–19.

Simpson, A., Reynolds, L., Light, I. and Attenborough, J. (2008) Talking with the experts: evaluation of an online discussion forum with mental health service users and student nurses. *Nurse Education Today*, **28**, 633–640.

Simpson, D., Fincher, R.M.E., Hafler, J.P. *et al.* (2007) *Advancing Edcators and Education: Defining the Components and Evidence of Educational Scholarship*, Association of American Medical Colleges, Washington, DC.

Sirianni, C. and Friedland, L. (2001) *Civic Innovation in America: Community Empowerment, Public Policy, and the Movement for Civic Renewal*, University of Claifornia Press, Berkeley.

Siwe, K., Wijma, B. and Bertero, C. (2006) 'A stronger and clearer perception of self'. Women's experience of being professional patients in teaching the pelvic examination: A qualitative study. *BJOG An International Journal of Obstetrics and Gynaecology*, **113**, 890–895.

Skills for Health (2006) You Can Influence the Quality of Healthcare Education, Skills for Health, Leeds.

Skinner, B.F. (1957) *Verbal Learning*, Appleton-Century-Crofts, New York.

Snow, D. and Benford, R. (1988) Ideology, frame resonance and participant mobilization. *International Social Movement Research*, **1**, 197–219.

Spandler, H. (2004) Friend or Foe? Towards a critical assessment of direct payments. *Critical Social Policy*, **24**(2), 187–209.

Spandler, H. (2006) *Asylum to Action: Paddington Day Hospital, Therapeutic Communities and Beyond*, Jessica Kingsley Publications, London.

Spandler, H. and Heslop, P. (2007) Exercising choice and control: independent living, direct payments and self harm, in *Beyond Fear and Control: Working with Young People Who Self Harm* (eds H. Spandler and S. Warner), PCCS books, Ross-on-Wye, Herefordshire, UK.

Spandler, H. and McKeown, M. (2008) Shifting Identities in a Context of Community Engagement and Commitments to Social Change. Academic Identities in Crisis Conference, 4–6 September 2008, University of Central Lancashire, Preston.

Spear, R. and Bidet, E. (2005) Social enterprise for work integration in 12 European countries: a descriptive analysis. *Annals of Public and Cooperative Economics*, **76**(2), 195–231.

Spencer, J., Blackmore, D., Heard, S. *et al.* (2000) Patient-oriented learning: a review of the role of the patient in the education of medical students. *Medical Education*, **34**, 851–857.

Stacy, R. and Spencer, J. (1999) Patients as teachers: a qualitative study of patients' views on their role in a community-based undergraduate project. *Medical Education*, **33**, 688–694.

Steffen, S. and Fothergill, A. (2009) 9/11 Volunteerism: a pathway to personal healing and community engagement. *The Social Science Journal*, **46**, 29–46.

Stevens, S. and Tanner, D. (2006) Involving service users in the teaching and learning of social work students: reflections on experience. *Social Work Education*, **25**, 360–371.

Swain, J., French, S. and Cameron, C. (2003) *Controversial Issues in a Disabling Society*, Open University Press, Maidenhead.

Sweeney, A., Beresford, P., Faulkner, A. *et al.* (2009) *This is Survivor Research*, PCCS Books, Ross-on-Wye, Herefordshire, UK.

Symon, A. and Dobb, B. (2008) An exploratory study to assess the acceptability of an antenatal quality-of-life instrument (the Mother-generated Index). *Midwifery*, **24**(4), 442–450.

Tarrow, S. (1998) *Power in Movement: Social Movements, Collective Action and Politics*, 2nd edn, Cambridge University Press, Cambridge.

Tew, J. and Hendry, S. (2003) User involvement in education and training in the West Midlands, mental health in higher education. http://www.mhhe.ltsn.soton.ac.uk/news/tew.asp (accessed November 2007).

Tew, J., Gell, C. and Foster, F. (2004) A Good Practice Guide. Learning from Experience. Involving Service Users and Carers in Mental Health Education and Training, Mental Health in Higher Education/NIMHE, Nottingham.

Tewksbury, L., English, R., Christy, C. *et al.* (2009) Scholarship of Application: When Service is Scholarship – A Workshop for Medical Educators. MedEdPORTAL: http://services.aamc.org/30/mededportal/servlet/s/segment/mededportal/?subid=7734 (accessed 5 January 2010).

Touraine, A. (1978) *The Voice and the Eye: An Analysis of Social Movements*, Cambridge University Press, Cambridge.

Towers, B. (1996) Health care and the new managerialism: policy, planning and organisation, in *Sociology: Insights in Health Care* (ed. A. Perry), Arnold, London.

Towle, A. and Goldolphin, W. (2008) Patient Involvement in Health Professional Education: A Bibliography, 1975–2008, Division of Health Care Communication, University of British Columbia.

Tritter, J., Daykin, N., Evans, S. and Sanidas, M. (2004) *Improving Cancer Services Through Patient Involvement*, Radcliffe Medical Press, Oxon.

Tukey, J.W. (1977) *Exploratory Data Analysis*, Addison-Wesley, London.

Turner, M. and Beresford, P. (2005) Contributing on Equal Terms: Service User Involvement and the Benefit System, Social Care Institute for Excellence, London, UK.

Turner, P., Sheldon, F., Coles, C. *et al.* (2000) Listening to and learning from the family carer's story: an innovative approach in interprofessional education. *Journal of Interprofessional Care*, **14**(4), 387–395.

Tyler, G. (2006) Addressing barriers to participation: service user involvement in social work training. *Social Work Education*, **4**, 385–392.

UNISON (2008) National Branch Seminar. Strategic Influence and Community Campaigning. Seminar Report, 22 May 2008, Unison, London.

Voronka, J., Frazee, C., Panitch, J., and Church, K. (2007) Shall We Chronicle? Storying 'Art with Attitude', Ryerson-RBC Institute for Disability Studies Research and Education, Toronto.

Wadsworth, Y. (1998) What is participatory action research? Action Research International. Paper 2. http://www.scu.edu.au/schools/gcm/ar/ari/p-ywadsworth98.html (accessed 9 January 2010).

Warne, T. and McAndrew, S. (2007) Passive patient or engaged expert? Using a Ptolemaic approach to enhance mental health nurse education and practice. *International Journal of Mental Health Nursing*, **16**, 224–229.

Werner, E. and Smith, R. (1982) *Vulnerable but Invincible: A Longitudinal Study of Resilient Children and Youth*, McGraw-Hill, New York.

Whelan, J. and Lyons, K. (2005) Community engagement or community action: choosing not to play the game. *Environmental Politics*, **14**, 596–610.

Whittaker, K. and Taylor, J. (2004) Learning from the experience of working with consumers in educational developments. *Nurse Education Today*, **24**, 530–537.

WHO (1948) Preamble to the Constitution of the World Health Organization as adopted by the International Health Conference, New York, 19–22 June 1946, and entered into force on 7 April 1948. Available at: http://www.who.int/bulletin/bulletin_board/83/ustun11051/en/ (accessed 14 August 2009).

Wieviorka, M. (2005) After new social movements. *Social Movement Studies*, **4**(1), 1–19.

Williamson, C. (2008) The patient movement as an emancipation movement. *Health Expectations*, **11**, 102–112.

Wills, J. (2007) Low pay, no way. *Red Pepper*, 155 (September), 20–27.

Wills, J. and Simms, M. (2004) Building reciprocal community unionism in the UK. *Capital and Class*, **82**(Spring), 59–84.

Winter, A., Wiseman, J. and Muirhead, B. (2006) University-community engagement in Australia: practice, policy and public good. *Education, Citizenship and Social Justice*, **1**(3), 211–230.

Wood, J. and Wilson-Barnett, J. (1999) The influence of user involvement on the learning of mental health nursing students. *Nursing Times Research*, **4**, 257.

Woodall, J. (1996) Managing culture change: can it ever be ethical. *Personnel Review*, **25**(6), 26–40.

Woodward, C.A. (1988) Questionnaire construction and question writing for research in medical education. *Medical Education*, **22**, 347–363

WHO (World Health Organisation) (1987) Learning together to work together for health, technical report No. 769. WHO, Geneva.

Wykurz, G. and Kelly, D. (2002) Learning in practice – developing the role of patients as teachers: literature review. *British Medical Journal*, **325**, 818–821.

Yuill, C. (2005) Marx: Capitalism, alienation and health. *Social Theory and Health*, **3**, 126–143.

Zigmond, A.S. and Snaith, R.P. (1983) The hospital anxiety and depression scale. *Acta Psychiatrica Scandinavica*, **67**(6), 361–370.

Zografos, C. (2007) Rurality discourses and the role of the social enterprise in regenerating rural Scotland. *Journal of Rural Studies*, **23**, 38–51.

APPENDICES

Appendix 1: Research and Evaluation Planning Worksheet

Research or Evaluation Team: Which teachers, service users, carers, learners and community members have a special interest in our project? Who should we recruit to ensure that all groups with an interest in this work are represented?_____

_____

_____

Research Question: Choose a topic and question that is important to educators, service users, carers, learners and/or others who care about your programme._____

_____

_____

Domains to Study or Evaluate:
Choose the domains that apply to this project and write a brief description of which aspects the project will study or evaluate.

_____ Process evaluation (Did we accomplish what we set out to do?): _____

_____

_____

_____ Satisfaction and other responses of participants:_____

_____

_____

_____ Impact of patients and families on the learners:_____

_____

_____

_____ Impact of involvement in health professional education on the service users, carers and other faculty:_____

_____

_____ Impact of service users' and carers' involvement in health professional education on healthcare:_____

_____

_____ Impact on communities through patients and families, faculty, advocacy groups and learners: _____

Research or Evaluation Design: The design that best fits our question is

_____ Audit or process evaluation

_____ Descriptive study with qualitative data

_____ Descriptive study with quantitative data

_____ Descriptive study with both qualitative and quantitative data

_____ Study to test an intervention with qualitative data

_____ Study to test an intervention with quantitative data

_____ Study to test an intervention with both qualitative and quantitative data

Data Collection:

How can we best work together as a team to design and implement data collection strategies?

How can we build valid observation tools, interview and focus group guides, or other data collection tools?

_____ Review the literature. What kind of literature?

_____

_____ Consult experts. Who? _____

_____

_____ Involve different members of our study team. Who will do what? How will we decide?_____

_____

What method(s) of data collection would best help answer our question? What could be done specifically within our context/limitations/institution?

_____ Observation (Watch people in the setting where the things we want to study happen.)

_____ Interviews (Ask questions of one or two people at a time, by phone or in person.)

_____ Focus groups (Ask questions of groups of 4–10 people, with opportunity for conversation in the group.)

_____ Document analysis (Review study reports, archives, minutes of meetings, diaries and other written records.)

_____ Paper- or computer-based questionnaires or surveys

_____ Other ways of gathering data:_____

_____

Data Management:

What data will we collect?

_____

What system can be put in place to keep track of data and make it easy to analyse?

_____

_____

What should be done to ensure that future replication of data collection and analysis is possible?

_____

Who will be responsible for collecting, managing, analysing data?

_____

What resources do we need?

Team Management:
How will we determine how often to have meetings and who should attend in order to have a smoothly functioning research team?

How will we address challenges?

Data Analysis/Interpretation:
Who will perform analysis/interpretation?

How can we improve the validity of the analysis?
_____ Collect data from several sources?
_____ Check back with learners, service users, carers or other faculty?
_____ Build in a process for reflection?
_____ Get expert help with statistics?
_____ Get expert help with qualitative analysis?
What specifically can we do to analyse our data?

_____

Review, Interpret, Summarize and Present the Data:
Who will be on the data review and interpretation team?

Who will be responsible for writing about the educational evaluation or research study?

_____

How will the results be presented and to whom?

_____

How will we evaluate the impact of our presentation on those we had hoped to influence?

_____

How will we take the results generated by the study and the impact of our presentation and plan next steps?

_____

Appendix 2: Terms of Reference for Comensus Advisory Group

As agreed at the inaugural meeting on 17 March 2004

Members of the Comensus Advisory Group will:

(i) Work to an ethos of cooperation and consensus to ensure that staff and students of UCLan's Faculty of Health fully engage with service users and carers in the four aspects of the Faculty business (education, research, practice and consultancy), in order to enhance skills, knowledge and employability.

(ii) Assure, by posing challenging questions, that the project aims and objectives are clear and that the project itself remains meaningful, systematic, comprehensive and sustainable whilst simultaneously keeping to timetable.

(iii) Advise on methods of engaging 'harder to reach' groups, action planning processes and training requirements or provision of training for service users.

(iv) Report on the Group's activities to the Faculty Executive Team and to receive reports from this team.

(v) Inform the project of relevant community activities and resources.

(vi) Consider matters relating to the project's accessibility and cultural sensitivity.

(vii) Establish dispute and conflict management processes.

(viii) Ensure that the social firm adopts a progressive model of employment and that any involvement of service users or carers during the development of the project is not merely tokenistic.

Appendix 3: Year One Issues and Solutions

Issues	Solutions
Representativeness Discussion about the relative contribution of community organization workers, individual service users and carers and professionals.	There would not be any expectation of representativeness from individual members of the CIT. They would be free to bring forward collective views, for example if they had affiliations to a wider group, but this would not be insisted upon. Individual experiences were to be valued. Workers from community groups/statutory sector organizations expected to bring institutional perspectives.
Payments Rates for payment and methods of accessing expenses and payment, especially for those on state benefits.	Service users: All individuals to be offered confidential welfare rights advice prior to accepting monies from the project. All out-of-pocket expenses (including travel, subsistence, substitute carers, etc.) paid in full, typically in cash. For CIT business: Monthly reimbursement of £35 unreceipted expenses, reflecting the demands placed upon participants in the project (cheques via university payroll). This amount can be paid directly to a local community group if people wish, or individuals can choose not to claim altogether. Discrete contributions over and above routine CIT work (teaching sessions, research consultancies) are agreed with particular budget holders. Advisory Group (AG) members from voluntary sector receive £50 per meeting attended in compensation for their time, paid to the organization not the individuals. All other AG members are not paid anything.
Inclusion Issues around inclusion, such as the language used, the presentation of documents and minutes (font size, pictures, style).	For launch event: supporters for service user attendees; post-it notes for people (or their supporters) to write down things they did not feel able to say; the use of cards that could be held up to stop the conversation if someone wanted to say something. Flip charts were left on walls. Font for all documents: ariel 12pt, double spaced, use of pictures, simple language

Issues	Solutions
Redirection of resources The redirection of resources to the community, for example in terms of meeting venues and provision of refreshments.	There is a commitment to share meetings between community venues and university rooms. When meetings are in the community local groups provide the catering. Big events, Summer Fairs for instance, are held in the community and any monies raised are redistributed back to the community. Relevant training for the CIT was to be purchased from appropriate community sources.
Complementary expertise The need to recognise complementary expertise between all the participating individuals.	Participants from all backgrounds have different starting levels of confidence and different talents and expertise. Support, training and capacity building will be provided. Resources to this effect within the AG were mobilised by the construction of a skills database identifying individuals and groups associated with specific forms of expertise.
Management of meetings Need to run meetings to time, respect outside commitments and allow space for all to speak.	Chair of meeting gradually taken over by Advisory Group (and later CIT) members. Agenda agreed by all in advance. System of yellow and red cards used to indicate when people wanted to speak. Agreement about the need to balance everyone's opportunity to speak with the need to finish on time.

Adapted from Downe *et al.*, 2007: 398.

Appendix 4: Terms of Reference for CIT

The Community Involvement Team (CIT) is at the centre of the Comensus project. It is the primary focus of user and carer involvement within the Comensus project and has primacy over other groups and meetings that arise in Comensus. The CIT is supported by the Comensus Advisory Group (name may change) but is free to accept or reject any such advice or support that is offered.

Our Community Involvement Team aims to influence training, research and development within the Faculty of Health by presenting our views and experiences and perspectives in ways that reflect, inform, share, champion and focus on promoting excellence in health and social care services.

We aim to do this in mutually supportive and respective relationships and partnerships.

The Community Involvement Team exists to:

- Influence strategic decision making in the Faculty of Health.
- Inform debate about best practice in involving users and carers in education, be directly involved in specific teaching and learning initiatives, and to promote and facilitate wider user and carer involvement. This to include face-to-face teaching, development of courses and learning materials, and involvement in all aspects of learning support and organization, such as validation and accreditation processes, marking and moderation, and so on.
- Inform debate about best practice in involving users and carers in research, be directly involved in specific research projects, and to promote and facilitate wider user and carer involvement. This to include involvement at all stages of the research process.
- Respond to requests from faculty staff or teams for specific examples of involvement (i.e. to either identify who might fulfil a contribution from within the CIT or wider groups affiliated to the project).
- Provide a link between the university and the community of Preston.
- Promote reciprocal practices and services between the community of Preston and the university – promoting goodwill and involvement at all levels.

We are committed to:

- Supporting each other.

- Addressing our own training and support needs.
- Extending our influence beyond this university into other centres of learning locally, nationally and internationally.
- Adopting such campaigns as are relevant to our aims but which do not detract from our main purpose.
- Informing ourselves of current practice within the university in order to identify gaps in learning and to develop a model for learning that is enhanced by user and carer experience and expertise.
- Question the basis of all work within the Faculty. To come up with new starting points, new conclusions.
- Developing the idea of the social firm to take forward the expertise of service users and carers in packages of training and consultancy to meet the needs of the Faculty of Health and other organizations.

Decision Making in the CIT

We expect most decisions to be taken after inclusive discussions between members. Ideally the work of the CIT will proceed on the basis of consensus decision making. When this is not possible a vote will take place and decisions will be made on the basis of simple majority. A quorum of 40% of eligible CIT members (eight individuals) will be necessary for meetings. UCLan personnel and Advisory Group representatives do not count for purposes of reaching quorum.

Care will be taken in discussions to make sure that:

- All views and contributions are respected and valued.
- Where there are different viewpoints brought forward from particular standpoints or, for example, between user and carer perspectives, efforts will be made to include the diversity of views in any CIT advice or report.

CIT Sub-groups

Work to inform discussions and decision making may be undertaken in the first instance by smaller groups of members in sub-groups.

The CIT may reserve decision making authority to the full CIT meetings, or delegate decision making to the most appropriate sub-group. To allow for all CIT members to be able to contribute to important decisions, in the first instance it will be taken that decision making is usually reserved to the full CIT. All sub-groups will report back to full CIT meetings. Devolution of decision making to sub-groups will only occur if it proves too difficult to take action or make progress between full CIT meetings.

Links to Comensus Advisory Group

The Advisory Group is made up of various representatives of key stakeholder organizations in the voluntary and statutory sector. It exists to support the Comensus project and helped in setting up the CIT.

Two members of the Advisory Group attend CIT meetings.

Advisory Group members can also be invited to assist CIT members with subgroup activities.

There is the facility to establish ad hoc groups which bring together Advisory Group and CIT membership.

Frequency of Meetings

The CIT aims to meet eleven times per year (with no meeting in August).

Alternate meetings are:

(a) Full CIT meetings.
(b) Meetings which are mostly taken up with activity in the sub-groups with everyone coming together as full CIT before and after the sub-group work.

Membership

The overall membership of the CIT will always attempt to be as inclusive as possible of a diverse range of user and carer perspectives and the range of user and carer perspectives covered by the work of the Faculty of Health.

Membership is for a fixed-term period of four years with an option to apply for one- or two-year extensions up to a maximum of six years in total. On a three-year cycle, one-third of the CIT membership will be renewed annually. This process will commence at the time when all of the initial CIT have completed four years in membership. From there on in new members will be eligible for renewal after four years in membership.

Recruitment of new members and replacement of members who leave will always be done in a way that seeks to achieve a balance of experienced members and new members in the CIT.

Membership of the CIT is by application only. Future application to the CIT will be managed by a specially constituted selection panel, which will be a combined sub-group of both Advisory Group and CIT.

Relationship with the Faculty Executive Team (FET)

The Faculty Executive Team is the management group in the Faculty of Health. It includes senior managers such as the heads of department and the Dean of the Faculty. It was this group that made the decision to allocate funds to provide for the Comensus project.

The CIT will develop communications and links with the FET:

- Comensus project coordinator will be briefed to carry business to the FET meetings.
- A delegate from the CIT will attend FET meetings as routine, and will be supported by the project coordinator.
- FET takes CIT business as standing item.
- CIT produces regular reports for FET (with assistance of project coordinator).
- FET delegate attends CIT meetings and is accountable for taking forward CIT initiated business in FET meetings.

Appendix 5: COMENSUS: Action Plan 2009

Quality Assurance Work Plan

AIM: To provide evidence of the value of our work to commissioners of Comensus and commit to continuous quality improvement.

Objective	By Whom	How	Timescale
To identify a sample of members from both CIT and Advisory Groups to undertake consultation exercise re the quality of our service	Project coordinator	• Annual focus group for Advisory Group • Quality circles twice a year for CIT • Use ladder of involvement, track changes	Annually Every six months
To ask service users individually for their views	Project coordinator	• Project coordinator will meet with new CIT members as part of induction process • Project coordinator will gain feedback as part of ongoing work • Project coordinator will interview each CIT member annually	Ongoing
To gather third party feedback wherever possible, that is, from academics, professionals	Project coordinator	• Send out questionnaire to third party when appropriate • Evaluate all training delivered	Ongoing
To ensure service user feedback is given to the Advisory Group, working group, Faculty Executive Team	Project coordinator Advisory Group/CIT liaison representatives	• Report to the associated groups, every three months • Write regular reports for presentation at Faculty Executive group • Act on feedback where appropriate • Have CIT representation in management meetings • Improve lines of communication with higher management	Every three months

Marketing Work Plan

AIM: To identify where our services are most needed and how we can raise our profile in these areas.

Objective	By Whom	How	Timescale
To further develop appreciation amongst academics, students and professionals we work with about our role and what is understood by the terms 'service user involvement' and Comensus	Project coordinator and CIT members	• Conduct a mail shot to individuals/local groups including Introductory letter and information pack.	End December 2009
		• Conduct minimum of three road shows on involving service users and carers in education to various academics. If successful exercise, roll out across the area and with other groups, for example National Health Service Trusts.	December 2009
		• Raise profile of project with students via student liaison office.	December 2009
		• Produce series of articles for publication including Involve and UCLan newsletters (PULSE and PLUTO) as well as academic journals.	December 2009
		• Build links with Primary Care Trusts and local hospitals	
To research demand for service user involvement within the Faculty of Health	Project coordinator and Faculty Lead for service user and carer involvement	• Update mapping exercise to identify gaps in current provision.	Ongoing
		• Market and promote our service to academics we are not currently reaching.	
		• Ensure activity is planned and that demand does not exceed resources	
Raise profile of Comensus with local service users and the wider community	Project coordinator, CIT and Advisory Groups	• Liaise with local service user and community groups.	Ongoing
		• Devise strategy for raising profile with service users and community	

Objective	By Whom	How	Timescale
Use proactive approach to develop Comensus within the Faculty of Health	Project coordinator and CIT team	• Market and promote the project brand, apply for awards. • Raise profile by introducing the project to academic staff, department heads. • Target academics who do not use the project currently, identify gaps. • Introduce project to university as a whole	Ongoing
Ensure the project is accessible	Project coordinator, and working group. Advisory Group	• Ensure all literature is produced in large fonts using easy words and pictures. • Ensure all venues are accessible. • Ensure we are aware of individuals support needs. • Update and promote Web site, add links. • CIT members to mentor new members. • Continue to address car parking	Ongoing
Produce service user led DVD on experiences of health and social care	CIT and community facilitated by coordinator	• Liaise with Marketing department and media studies over facilities available. • Recruit people to be involved. • Identify independent funding if needed. • Put on Web site	December 2009
Produce first draft of Book	Book steering group, Soo Downe, Mick McKeown and project coordinator	• Collaborative book reflecting on the experience of developing the project. • Identify possible funding	March 2009
Celebrate the successful formation of the CIT with the community and Faculty	CIT members, staff, advisory group	• Host awareness raising event of Comensus. • Raise profile at various community events. • Invite vice chancellor to CIT meeting. • Apply for national awards. • Display movable boards	December 2009

Develop Core Work

AIM: To ensure our core work is carried out efficiently

Objective	By Whom	How	Timescale
Support the CIT group and its associated sub-groups	Project coordinator, Mick McKeown and project administrator	• Ensure regular minutes and agendas are produced. • Ensure the power of the project lies with the CIT. • Service the meetings. • Act on decisions taken. • Report and give feedback to CIT group. • Ensure good communication between CIT and Advisory Group. • Pay expenses. • Ensure all members supported. • Ensure members offered welfare rights appointments. • Provide training for CIT members. • Explore with university what the CIT can be offered for involvement other then monetary gain. • Develop the skills of CIT members so they will independently run and manage their own sub-group meetings.	Ongoing
Support the Advisory Group	Project coordinator, Mick McKeown and project administrator	• Ensure regular minutes and agendas are produced. • Service the meetings. • Act on decisions taken. • Report and give feedback to Advisory Group. • Ensure good communication between CIT and Advisory Group, hold joint meeting.	Ongoing
Liaise and support research endeavour attached to project	Project coordinator, Mick McKeown and research group	• Participate with and support research activities. • Maintain good channels of communication between all project partners. • Support research papers sub-group reflecting on the messages we wish to put out to the wider audience. • Ensure those academics who have no funds for involvement contribute to writing papers, and so on. • Support Three Keys for Mental Health user-led bid	Ongoing

Objective	By Whom	How	Timescale
Ensure policies and procedures are adhered to and project specific policies developed and reviewed regularly	Project coordinator and working group	• Review UCLan's policies ensuring the following are developed by the project if required. • Equal opportunities. • Recruitment and selection. • Training. • Volunteer Policy. • Confidentiality. • Access to information. • Build into quality assurance system	Ongoing
Ensure all paperwork reflects university standards	Project coordinator, CIT members	• Review paperwork regularly.	Ongoing
Become a central resource for service user activity across the Faculty of Health	CIT and working group	• Market and promote Comensus. • Support and develop service user activity across the Faculty. • Develop a Faculty wide service user involvement strategy and payment strategy. • Write good practice guidelines for service user/carer involvement. • Attract new members for new Advisory Group	Ongoing December 2009
Meet regularly with commissioners and other stakeholders to review the service	Project coordinator Project Team Management Group	• Build in review of service every three to six months	Ongoing
Continue to grow involvement opportunities	Everyone	• Market, promote and use all opportunities to develop and increase our place as an important part of the Faculty • Ensure involvement is systematic and integrated	Ongoing
Identify and consolidate project funding	Comensus team	• Consolidate Faculty funding. • Apply for independent funding for project.	Ongoing

Research

AIM: To evaluate the process and outcomes of the project, and to contribute to its development through the action research project.

Objective	By Whom	How	Timescale
To ensure that participants views are fed into the development of the project	Project coordinator	Regular group and individual interviews	Ongoing
To ensure that project participants contribute to research design	Project coordinator	Discussion at Advisory and CIT groups	At least at every other CIT/Advisory Group meeting
To map service user involvement in the Faculty of Health	Project coordinator	Regular mapping exercises. Update School of Nursing Good Practice Guidelines	Ongoing
To ensure that the project is up to date with relevant existing and newly emerging literature	Project coordinator	Read widely and keep up to date with new initiatives	Ongoing
Within the available budget to pursue additional lines of enquiry as they arise	Research coordinator. Project coordinator	Sub-studies of various designs as appropriate	Depends on sub-study
To support project participants where they wish to engage in research activity	Research coordinator. Project coordinator	• By ensuring that interest in undertaking research is regularly sought • By allocating a member of the project team to any individual/group who wants to help with research work	During every CIT meeting. When interest is expressed
To report on progress regularly	Research coordinator. Project coordinator	• Feedback at working group, advisory and CIT meetings • Interim report for relevant heads of school and Dean	Ongoing. Annually by January each year
To disseminate the findings of the project	Research coordinators Project coordinator CIT	• Articles for local press • Journal articles • Conference presentations • Feedback on Web site • Maximise CIT contributions to published output	Ongoing

Attract outside funding and develop a body of work.

Objective	By Whom	How	Timescale
Complete innovation in participation lesson plans	CIT and Project coordinator	• Hold a number of focus groups and develop lesson plans collaboratively with service users and carers	January 2009
Sandbox – action research to develop peer-to-peer support within service user and carer groups	Mick McKeown and Sandbox staff and community members	• Hold a number of focus groups with interactive technology to develop support mechanisms collaboratively with service users and carers	December 2009
Bradton – develop a Web-based virtual community	Bradford university, Mick McKeown and community members	• Develop a virtual community based on real-life experiences including a virtual voluntary sector	Ongoing
Develop Skills for Care Strategic Forum	Comensus Coordinator	• Develop a strategic forum for Skills for Care Hold a number of focus groups Set up systems for involvement	March 2009
Develop and host the second Authenticity to Action Conference	CIT and staff	• Develop a planning committee • Invite people to present their work • Obtain sponsorship • Invite participants • Hold the conference • Review event	November 2009

Support SUCAG and social work activities

Objective	By Whom	How	Timescale
Support SUCAG	Project coordinator and project administrator	• Ensure regular minutes and agendas are produced • Service the meetings • Act on decisions taken • Report and give feedback to Head of Social Work. • Pay expenses • Ensure all members are supported • Ensure members offered welfare rights appointments • Provide training for SUCAG members • Explore with university what SUCAG can be offered for involvement other then monetary gain • Develop the skills of SUCAG members so they will independently run and manage their own group meetings • Write regular reports • Monitor and review budget regularly • Support and supervise project administrator	Ongoing
Support Congresses	Project coordinator and project administrator	• Liaise with academic staff re development and running of Congresses • Liaise with local community groups re involvement • Support community members to run own workshops • Develop all admin materials, for example poster, door signs, signing sheets, evaluations • Support service users/carers to plan opening address and closure of the congresses • Review evaluations and write report	Ongoing
Liaise and support partner colleges	Project coordinator	• Maintain good channels of communication between all project partners • Support partner colleges to engage with service users and carers	Ongoing

Appendix 6: Year Three Sub-Groups of The Community Involvement Team

Knowledge Support Sub-group

Set up to develop good practice guidelines for academics. Designed 'involving service users and carers' and 'involving service users and carers in research' booklets. Developed an internal skills directory outlining expertise of advisory group members and a small database outlining Community Involvement Team (CIT) members' and other contacts' health and caring experiences.

Leaflets and Language Sub-group

Set up to ensure that documents developed by Comensus used accessible language, easy words and pictures, and did not contain jargon. The group also helped academics with their documents, so that items for community distribution were prepared in simpler formats. Its members also helped develop and maintain the Web site, a process for developing resources within the Faculty and information for a mental health consultation event.

Research Sub-group

This Group looked at engaging with academic researchers on the development of academic papers, conference presentations and future research activity. It also focused on raising awareness of service user and carer involvement in research with other academics. It worked closely in partnership with academics who acted as mentors.

Ethics Sub-group

This sub-group focused on current ethical issues and wider debate, examined the complexities of health and social care and ensured this was on the agenda across the faculty.

Strategy Sub-group

Set up to examine the progress, development and direction of service user and carer involvement in the faculty; this group planned strategic activity and action.

Social Firm Sub-group

This group concentrated on developing an independent social firm to take forward the work of Comensus. It carried out related marketing, planning and research activity.

Appendix 7: Year 3 Issues and Solutions

Issues	Solutions
Communication barriers	• CIT developed good practice guidelines for involving service users and carers and accessible writing guide. • Academics constantly reminded about the use of jargon and acronyms. Chairs of all academic meetings asked to remind staff before meeting starts not to use jargon. • Standing representative assigned to some groups to support other CIT members who were new to the group and act as mentor.
Tokenism	• Coordinator and CIT members actively promoted strategic involvement as the way forward and planned activity accordingly. • Where teaching involvement only requested, promoted service user and carer involvement across modules as good practice. • Used academic champions to promote service user and carer involvement in to a variety of arenas. • Highlighted advantage of service user and carer involvement as added 'value' to activities within faculty. • Raised awareness of good practice within divisions.
Strain of involvement	• Provided comprehensive package of training for all CIT members. • Coordinator and other staff members supported CIT members on an individual basis providing 'coaching' and support. • CIT and Advisory Group focused on the bigger picture – what we were trying to achieve. • Group moved beyond functional and became one where people supported each other, socialised and were kind to each other.
Representativeness	• At initial meetings the Advisory Group and CIT decided not to be sidetracked by this debate as it detracts from their endeavours. Members are recruited because they themselves have had experience of health and social care or care for someone who does. However, many of the CIT are members of other groups themselves and can express wider views within specific contexts, but there is no expectation that they must do so.

Issues	Solutions
	• We accepted that any group could not represent all sectors of the population and explain this clearly, however, when recruiting new members we try to ensure the group is diverse as possible.
	• We remind academics that they too are individuals who unless have carried out extensive research or consultation cannot possibly speak for their peers.
Culture	• Preparation for service users and carers is vital so they don't experience 'culture shock'.
	• Service users and carer involvement is promoted across the Faculty as being desirable and good practice by managers and Comensus academic champions.
	• Service users and carers supported in meetings with a remit agreed by all that asking questions does not make people 'stupid'.

Appendix 8: Protocol for the Development of Learning Resources Involving Service Users and/or Carers

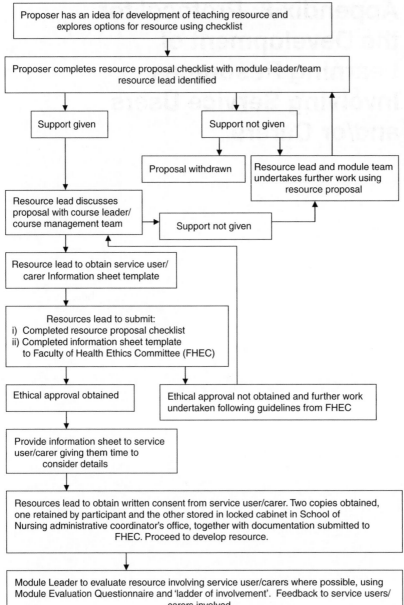

Proposer has an idea for development of teaching resource and explores options for resource using checklist

Proposer completes resource proposal checklist with module leader/team resource lead identified

Support given

Support not given

Proposal withdrawn

Resource lead and module team undertakes further work using resource proposal

Resource lead discusses proposal with course leader/ course management team

Support not given

Resource lead to obtain service user/ carer Information sheet template

Resources lead to submit:
i) Completed resource proposal checklist
ii) Completed information sheet template
    to Faculty of Health Ethics Committee (FHEC)

Ethical approval obtained

Ethical approval not obtained and further work undertaken following guidelines from FHEC

Provide information sheet to service user/carer giving them time to consider details

Resources lead to obtain written consent from service user/carer. Two copies obtained, one retained by participant and the other stored in locked cabinet in School of Nursing administrative coordinator's office, together with documentation submitted to FHEC. Proceed to develop resource.

Module Leader to evaluate resource involving service user/carers where possible, using Module Evaluation Questionnaire and 'ladder of involvement'. Feedback to service users/ carers involved.

Appendix 9: Service User/Carer/Public Consent Form

1. I .... (*print name of the person getting involved*) ('the Participant')
   of...
   ....
   ....*where you live*)
   will allow the information I have shared about myself to be held by the University of Central Lancashire (the "University") and used to make teaching and learning resource(s) as below:

   Photograph ☐

   Artwork ☐

   Video/DVD ☐

   Audio Recording ☐

   Text based Teaching and Learning Materials ☐

   Other (Please specify) ☐

   (Please tick the box/es which apply)

2. I have read (or have had read to me) and understand the information sheet about the teaching and learning materials.

3. I agree to this teaching and learning resource(s) being shared for education and training purposes with the following audiences and venues:

   • With students and staff in courses/workshops/conferences offered by the University of Central Lancashire ☐

   • In any health or social care education and training event to any audience occurring regionally/nationally/internationally ☐

   • In Problem Based/Open/Distance Learning Packages/DVD ☐

   (Please tick the box/es above which apply)

4. I understand that access to computer based teaching and learning materials, including video clips, used by staff and students are password protected.
5. I understand that health care professionals within the School of Nursing are guided by rules set by their professional organization (e.g. nurses – Nursing and Midwifery Council).
6. I understand that the material I have made and its use means that I may be recognised by staff and/or students.
7. I have been informed and agree that copyright and all other rights in the teaching and learning resource(s) are and will remain owned by the University.

> I have been told and agree that the teaching and learning materials produced will be owned by the University.

8. I understand that the resource made will be destroyed when it is no longer needed.
9. I agree to be part of the making of the teaching and learning materials and agree to undertake this role:

With payment (as agreed)   ☐

Without payment   ☐

(Please tick the box which applies)

10. I am aware and agree that I may withdraw my consent at any time until the teaching and learning resource(s) has been fully developed (and I have been given the opportunity to see it), after which time withdrawal of my consent will not be possible. (Requests for withdrawal should be in writing and sent to the School of Nursing, University of Central Lancashire, Preston PR1 2HE).

> I know and I am aware that I can change my mind at any time up until the material has been finished (I have been given the opportunity to see it), after which time I cannot change my mind. (To change my mind, I have to write to the University.)

I have read and understood the above information and terms, and give my agreement and permission as described above.

> I understand the information given to me and agree for the materials to be made and used as described above.

Additional Information *(if any)*:

Participant's signature. . . . .
Name of Participant. . . . .
Date. . . . .

(An advocacy worker/carer/health professional/key worker should sign below if the Participant is (due to inability to do so) unable to sign but has had the terms of this document explained to him or her and has indicated his/her informed consent).

I have explained the meaning of this document to the Participant to the best of my ability and in a way which I believe he/she has understood and I believe that he/she wishes to proceed:

Advocacy worker/carer/health professional/key worker
Signature. . . . .
Full Name . . . .
Position . . . .
Date . . . .

(Use the signature block below only where the participant is a service user/carer who is representing an organization, e.g. NHS Trust or Charity, and its consent is required)

I confirm that. . . . .*(name of organization)* consents to the participation of . . . .*(name of individual)* on the terms set out above.

Signature. . . . .
Full name . . . .
Position in the organization . . . .
Date . . . .

Index

Page numbers in *italics* represent figures, those in **bold** represent tables.